THE ART OF HEALTHY LIVING

*A Mind-Body Approach to Inner
Balance and Natural Vitality*

HOMAYOUN SADEGHI, M.D.

ISBN: 0996971300

ISBN 13: 9780996971300

Library of Congress Control Number: 2015917741

Weyburn & Wise Publishing

Printed in the United States of America

For information about special discounts available for bulk purchases, sales promotions, fundraising and educational needs, please visit www.SadeghiMD.com

Table of Contents

Dedication

Gathering a mere diary of the experiences I had humbly come across, I never imagined that may be someday I would actually share my thoughts. Now that I look back, I see that right from the start I had been laboring for you, the reader, with all my heart. Sharing my intimate insights and private thoughts confers an honor I would have never even remotely dreamed of. I hereby dedicate this book to you, my readers.

Acknowledgments

How can I possibly acknowledge every single person who has ultimately contributed to the knowledge base that's been laid out in this book? I've had the opportunity to learn from many teachers in the stream of life. Constructive or not, many of their teachings have been assimilated in my heart. My greatest thanks to those of you who have crossed my path.

The opportunity to write this book was a miracle that was made possible by the caring support of my parents, S. and M. Sadeghi. They provided a tremendous amount of support by being patient, believing in me, and offering an undying source of inspiration, encouragement, and love.

Introduction

This book highlights the delicate, interconnected nature of the mind and the body. It describes the intimate role the mind plays in maintaining a healthy body and proposes that every impulse generated in the mind may intimately affect the health of the body. It shows how by becoming conscious of this causal connection, you will realize that your state of health is highly dependent on the way your mind engages your body.

The crux of this book showcases the mind as the nurturing nest of the physical body. It encourages a culture of reliance on inner guidance, insight, and intuition to promote a healthy body. It inspires an inner journey to learn the wisdom that lies at the heart of the body.

Before embarking on this amazing inward journey, however, it's important to have a solid understanding of how the mind can ultimately help rejuvenate, balance, or inadvertently damage the body. Ordinarily, the human mind plays a key role in directing the vital force of life. On a subconscious level, it orchestrates and regulates the functions of life. When it's in tune with the melody that supports the force of life, it lets the body radiate with vitality and exude health.

Is your body vibrating with the sweet wonder of life? Are you inherently charged with feelings of energy and health? Are you in shape, fit, and glowing with the hues of life? Is there anything that's keeping you from living a balanced, healthy, or vibrant life? Physically, these states can never be reliably sustainable without harnessing the nurturing power of the creative mind.

Are you consciously aware of the dynamics that form the nucleus of your mind-body connection? Do you have an active role in mediating or influencing this connection? If not, wouldn't you want to understand and use the tremendous revitalizing power that lies at the core of this dynamic connection?

Health is not a product of chance at all; it takes effort, wisdom, and insight to understand the meaning and the mechanics of it all. Like the sun's rays, the elements of health and healing are abundant and available for us all. It's up to us to avail ourselves of them and to take advantage of them all.

Perhaps in order to better understand the nature and extent of this connection, it may be best to begin by identifying the core substance of your true self, by evaluating who or what you are. Are you the body? The mind? Or a higher entity that exists completely beyond the scope of a mere body or mind?

To honestly answer these questions, you must dare to delve deep within. You must rediscover and reestablish a conscious connection with that spark, which is the source of the creation of everything. You must find your role within that cosmic symphony that stretches across eternity and encompasses everything. You need to know your own place and status within the greater scheme of it all.

To be perfectly healthy, you must first connect with that higher self, which intuitively guides us all. You need to know that you are an indivisible part of a greater all. Only then can you ever really hope to understand the concept and the determinants of health and healing at all.

It took me decades to understand the cause-and-effect relationship between one's inner thoughts and habits, and the quality of health. Even as a doctor, I was shocked to finally realize the critical role the mind plays in creating vitality, disease, aging, and health. In truth, I rarely considered the importance of mind as a fundamental determinant of health. Like pieces of a puzzle, however, everything simply fell in place when I finally learned to look within and discover the more subtle and deeper landscapes in life.

My teaching institutions were of world-class caliber

and exceptionally well rounded. Nevertheless, I found it difficult to find extra time to pause and reflect. In medical school, I was too busy learning the wealth of information that had ambushed me. I was drowning in demanding rotations and subjects like anatomy, pharmacology, pathology, and biochemistry. My postgraduate residency training emphasized hands-on proficiency by means of volume and breadth of pathology.

As I transitioned out of training, I began my career by serving as a university instructor. It wasn't until I became a private practitioner, however, that I began to put two and two together and noticed the abstract interplay between the mind and the body in creating energy, vitality, and healing.

Throughout the years that followed, my observations were slowly confirmed as I gained more insight and intuition, spurred on by an insatiable thirst for introspection and self-reflection. Little by little, the role of mind became increasingly evident as I supplemented my medical skills with intuitive knowledge and inner guidance.

What had been repeatedly emphasized in residency and medical school finally became clear: a loving smile, a helping hand, and a passionate display of compassion and care go a long way in healing a patient who's been lost in a hopeless despair. As you will see, the wealth of information in this book was not necessarily obtained by randomized trials or scientific experiments but rather from intuitive observations and relevant internal questions. Therefore, the standards in this book cannot necessarily all be gauged by scientific methods but rather by individual reflections and inner observations.

Here, you will find brief answers to many of the unanswered questions about life, disease, health, aging, and healing. But for many, these answers can at best only serve as clues in the process of health and healing. We humans all live on the same earthly plane, but we do not necessarily share the same level of understanding and insight about everything. While one may be rich in the culture of art and music, another may love history, engineering, or medicine, and have no taste or tolerance for any form of art or music.

Each and every one of us tends to be influenced by different ideas, histories, values, and experiences. Regardless of age, color, sex, or cultural differences, the diversity of experiences among us is beyond conception. Therefore, what may be easily comprehensible to one may seem obscure and require years of explanation and training for another. In light of this, though the simple knowledge contained in this book may help you heal your wounds and regain your health and state of youth, without the right understanding, it would be childish to rely on it as the sole means of achieving recovery and physical healing.

You can certainly register an eight-year-old in a college course, but you can't expect her to have a complete understanding of the information she takes away from that course. It often takes years to internalize and assimilate knowledge from the inside out. Therefore, for an ill-stricken novice, it would be wise to use this information as a supplement, not as a comprehensive means of treatment. In time, with practice, you will gain more insight and learn to heal yourself from the inside out. But until then it is best to do what currently needs to be done.

Throughout this book, I tend to use key terms to drive home certain concepts, in hopes of highlighting the most overlooked yet crucial elements of the mind-body dynamics. To the casual reader, these concepts may seem rather obvious, but for the young at heart, they form the basis upon which they can reliably learn to grow and evolve in this world.

The keynote of growth and advance in any subject is *practice*; practice is the breakfast of champions. It is an instrumental tool in reprogramming the subconscious mind to help you achieve favorable outcomes in life. The layered concepts outlined in this book are intended to do just that. It is my hope to serve by genuinely sharing the lessons and the experiences that have helped me grow in life.

CHAPTER 1

The Virtual Nature of the Universe

THIS IS ALL A DREAM

*I just woke up from a dream where
everything was so real.*

All the actors and the actresses seemed so real.

*I woke up startled, but suddenly the
truth flashed before me:*

This life is nothing but a projection of me.

I create all of this, simply to learn about me.

Everything in this life is for me; there
is no one else—it's all me.

I create a projection of this world solely for me.

Sleeping, dreaming, awake; these are
all external projections of me.

My father, my mother, my friends, and all that
surrounds me are nothing but a projection of me.

Realizing this, I finally understand that I need to be
kind to everyone, because everyone is a projection of me.

Everyone is a projection, created by me to learn about me.

Finally, I see that this whole universe and everything
in it are nothing but an extension of me.

Finally, I see that by interacting with others,
I am in truth learning to love me.

Henceforth, the more I learn about me, the more
my surroundings become harmonious for me.

Everything is a projection of me to learn about me.

The more I learn about me, the more I
see the truth that sets me free.

Now I see that all along, the whole time, everything
I have done and everything I have seen has been
nothing but a projection of me to learn about me.

There is no one else in this world but me; it's all about me.

This is all a drama I have created to learn about me.

I animate others to teach me about me.

*My wealth, my health, my house, my car, my
reach of influence, my behavior, and my social
interactions are all reflections of the depth
of the understanding I have about me.*

*When the light of truth finally shines on me, I begin
to realize that I am creating this world for me.*

*Then I realize that there is nothing to fear, because
this is all a projection of me to learn about me.*

*Whether awake or in a dream, what I am experiencing
is nothing but a projection of me to learn about me.*

*Knowing this, now I realize that I can instantly heal me,
I can instantly create a happy, healthy, and wealthy me.*

*I am the creator of my world; this world
is here for no one else but me.*

What a dream...

LIFE ON EARTH

Life on Earth is nothing but a captivating drama that serves to engage our emotions and stimulate our senses. Earth is nothing but a stage, a virtual deck on which we animate our desires and chase our dreams. It's a place where we can experiment with and test the outermost limits of our desires, emotions, and feelings.

This planet is a virtual battlefield created for us to mentally and spiritually evolve by engaging, challenging, and conquering our desires, emotions, and feelings. The very senses with which we experience our triumphs, our defeats, our uncertainties, our fears, our lusts, our greed, our angers, our demons, our sorrows, and our joys miraculously bind us to the delusions we experience on this earthly plane.

A Shift in Awareness

We rely on our sense perceptions to understand this world. The world we see, hear, touch, smell, and taste seems to be a solid representation of what we presume to be our entire universe. In reality, however, this palpable universe is nothing but a construct that is personalized to suit our core beliefs and embedded assumptions. We literally filter the world through our senses based on our teachings, beliefs, assumptions, and past experiences.

Our brains generally filter the world through the narrow perception of our five senses. This helps us focus so that we can make sense out of the unorganized chaos that imminently surrounds us. Without these filters, this world would be practically foreign to us.

Of course, this filtering process is subconsciously limited by the narrow confines of our own beliefs and life experiences. That's why at times our sense perceptions can easily fail us. As a matter of fact, we don't hesitate to doubt ourselves when, rightfully or not, others dare to take a stand and boldly challenge us.

Given the malleable nature of the human mind, it would be no surprise to think that we may have collectively adopted socially agreed-upon models and rules of how this world should be. In truth, what we call reality is only a model of perception, a tale, a point of reference that we have established arbitrarily.

Concepts like air travel or wireless technology, for example, were only but flashes of fantasy until we were able to fit them in our models of reality. We all know that only few centuries ago, the idea of the lifestyles we lead in today's world had no basis in reality.

We live in a fairy world, constructed by self-imposed models of virtual reality. Though as a race, we all collectively subscribe to what a model of reality should be, each and every one of us tends to settle into and experience a slightly different version of reality. Otherwise this world would be a boring place indeed. The nature of our homes, jobs, interactions, and relationships only testify to the level of understanding we have each reached in creating and glorifying our own personal realities.

What if your poverty is nothing but your own carelessly preconceived notion of what your financial state should be? What if your state of health conforms to your blind acceptance of how things should be? What if your happiness depends on money, relationships, predetermined results, and contingencies? Aren't you creating your own predefined version of reality?

Life is a game, a game of virtual reality. On Earth, each individual is by default an active participant in this game of virtual reality. A game, whether played on a computer, in an arena, or on a field, must by definition have rules and laws for its participants to engage in. Caught up in this drama, lost in this virtual maze, we misunderstand the rules, and therefore suffer the indignities of poverty, disease, discomfort, and insanity.

You are the creator of your universe. You are the choreographer, the actor, and the playwright of your own universe. If you but wake up and realize your mistake, you will have the potential to change your entire universe. You have every right to be healthy, you have the right to feel happy. You are entitled to be wealthy. Your only limit is your own level of flexibility, imagination, and creativity. Learn the rules; change your assumptions. Adopt empowering beliefs. Before you know it, this world will reshuffle itself to reflect your new assumptions and new beliefs.

EVERYTHING IS CONNECTED

Where do I stand in this vast realm of infinite design? I appear to have a mind filled with private thoughts, clothed with an isolated body, defined in space and time; yet I feel like I am an integral part of a bigger plan, a greater cause. I feel a peculiar sense of connection with everyone and everything around the world, one that transcends not only the boundaries of this planet but also those planets that lie far beyond my solar system, far beyond my puny cosmic hole.

Somehow I feel an invisible connection that extends far beyond the reach of my physical form. I feel it when my heart throbs in unison with the one I love. I share it with millions of others when I burst with pride as we land a discovery mission on Mars. I sense it when I feel disconsolate, watching others suffer halfway across the globe.

Somehow I find myself physically isolated and quarantined within the boundaries of my skin and bones, yet I feel connected and in touch with everyone and everything that is known or unknown. Is there an invisible link that collectively unites all individual souls?

At times, millions in the masses come together for a single cause. Some are touched by a common form of music, while others share a united view through politics, religion, science, or public laws. What is it that forms these invisible bonds when we all unite through a common interest, for a reason, or for a cause? All in all, there must be an instinctive state we all intuitively share in our hearts.

There must be a connecting link, an underlying medium that binds us all.

I have a physical body that I can see, hear, and touch, but I am also a spiritual being, an immaterial, intangible entity, filled with ethereal hopes, emotions, dreams, and thoughts. Although I work to make money and buy food, I find myself occasionally praying to a higher source, a connecting link, a motherly or fatherly figure to increase my income so that I can buy more food. Although I go to the doctor and rely on medications to heal my wounds, I find myself occasionally praying to a higher source to help speed up the healing of those wounds.

Although I try to put money aside for a rainy day, I feel urged to occasionally pray to a higher source and rely on my fate, in hopes that I may never have to see that day. Humankind has been around for millennia, yet I'm still unable to confidently say that there is someone or something out there that watches over me to save my day.

I'm torn between the hard choices I face: Which do I accept? The concrete, solitary life I find myself engaged in day by day? Or that ethereal connection I blindly rely on when I pray for things, things that are beyond my reach, far, far away?

Perhaps at a deeper level, every drop of creation in nature shares a common point of origin that binds every animate and inanimate manifestation of life to a common thread. Perhaps there is a primordial force that nourishes, sustains, and evolves the core substance of life itself. Perhaps, there is a starting point from which the scientifically theoretical "big bang" is assumed to have taken shape.

Perhaps, hidden in the background, there is a woven web that connects the ethereal realm of spirituality to the more tangible planes of physical reality. Perhaps this web supports earthly endeavors, while resting on the foundation of peace, faith, unity, love, beauty, and harmony. Oh, what we would possibly accomplish if we but knew that we could eternally draw from that communal web of information and energy collectively.

Decades ago, Albert Einstein coined the popular phrase "spooky action at a distance." His remark referred to a quantum theory concept the scientists call "entanglement." In layman's terms, entanglement tells the tale of how particles may be connected in a mysterious way, even when spatially separated. In other words, it describes how two distant tiny objects may affect each other, even though they may be light-years apart.

It's hard to account for such spontaneous connection when these objects may be galaxies apart. The sheer distance alone should automatically rule out any form of physical, chemical, or even wireless connection between the two. So then how do these two objects communicate simultaneously when they are so far apart?

Consider a hologram, which is nothing but a laser-aided, three-dimensional image. Holograms are interesting because they can be broken into pieces but still preserve the integrity of the original image in every single piece. In other words, every shredded piece of the photograph inherently projects the entire image, as if it were individually self-contained and completely whole.

This implies that every piece is literally one complete whole, even if you take one piece northward and another to the South Pole. Naturally, manipulating the image would affect all the other images as a whole.

This may shed light on how two tiny objects may be in tune with each other, without exchanging any cryptic signals, regardless of the distance between them. The seeming figment of separation between the two is really nothing but a grand illusion. The two distant objects that seem separate in your eyes are in truth inseparable aspects of one reality, one grand whole.

Humans on many occasions experience precipitous flashes of vision that provide sudden bits and pieces of information about others they may intimately know. We've all heard of twins occasionally saying the same thing or experiencing the same feeling at the same time, even if they live thousands of miles apart.

You begin to think of a loved one, when he or she suddenly picks up the phone to call you out of nowhere at all. A mother feels the pangs of pain in the pit of her stomach when her daughter feels the jolt of an earthquake somewhere in a distant land, oceans apart. Are these random incidences? Or are they just simple testimonial accounts of that subtle connection we all identify with deep in our hearts?

What is it that supports this connection? What else but that universal omnipresent source (call it energy, intelligence, or force) that permeates the vast realm of creation—the same fundamental source that bestirs all?

Science tells us that we are all made out of the same stuff. For example, although a crocodile and a monkey look and behave differently, the physical difference you perceive in their appearances is only skin-deep; it's only a mirage, an illusion—that's all.

In reality, they are not so different from each other after all. In truth, at a deeper level, they are almost identical. They are made out of the same elements that share a common lot.

On a subtler level, they are both made out of a conglomeration of individual cells that are confined in time and space. It's the intelligence and the order in which these cells and their constituents are put together that allows you to distinguish the appearance of one from the other—that's all.

When we look deeper, we see that the cells that make up their bodies are made out of the same identical molecules recycled from food, water, air, and other earthly stuff. These molecules are made up of atoms, and even more elementary yet, protons, electrons, and other subatomic particles that are basically finer constituents of life.

If we keep dissecting even further, we reach a certain point of existence where matter no longer stays confined within the boundaries of their bodies at all. At this level, some subatomic particles can randomly travel through solid objects and even penetrate the boundaries that separate the monkey from the crocodile. In other words, there is a point at which even matter itself is free from the illusion of individuality: the illusion that is falsely perceived by us.

At last, we see that in reality, we are all made out of the same earthly—or, more accurately, cosmic—stuff. Our bodies are literally bathing in a hodgepodge soup that is made out of the same atomic and subatomic ingredients that create the universe, the same building blocks of creation itself.

Like the fish in the sea, we live in a souplike ocean that contains all the primal ingredients needed for life. We have somehow managed to condense and mold little bits and clumps of this oceanic stuff into different bodies and shapes that make up the garden variety we see in life. Humans, elephants, zebras, monkeys, trees, plants, and worms are all different manifestations of the same primordial stuff.

Each condensed mold expresses its own unique individuality. Each mold possesses its own unique appearance, qualities, characteristics, and behaviors, yet it is animated by the same universal essence, the same animating force that encompasses everything.

By reason then, if we are all made out of the same fundamental elements that make up this cosmic, souplike stuff, we should know and feel every wave that ripples through it, should we not? We should be able to eavesdrop on every emotion, every affliction, and every behavior or action that is felt by others in this universal stuff, should we not?

In fact we do. Undeniably, at one point or another, we have all experienced some form of extrasensory perception, something that might have helped us avert danger or make the right decisions in life, have we not?

The reason we don't experience these moments more often is because we have completely shut ourselves out of the opportunity to accept anything beyond the narrow limits imposed by our rational minds. We have mindlessly chosen to rely on our traditional physical senses, as opposed to tuning into and connecting with our intuitive feelings and thoughts.

Intuitive feelings and thoughts can take shape in the form of visions, epiphanies, realizations, or just random, unsolicited thoughts. They help us draw sparks of wisdom when we by chance eavesdrop into the cosmic soup from which we all take part. When properly tuned into, they can lend a more instinctual understanding of the nature of our connection with the universal mind.

How do we strengthen this connection with the universal mind? Perhaps the answer lies in understanding that we are not outsiders trying to peek inside. Rather, we are simple extensions of the same primordial source that gives rise to the vast creation we see in life.

Like ice sculptures, we are carefully chiseled out of the same source that comes down as rain and fills our oceanic reservoirs. We are made out of the same ethereal stuff. We don't have to melt the ice to see the connection; we just have to remember who we are.

Looking at the concept of life in this light, we can finally see how we are not separate, isolated individuals, interacting in the game of life. Rather, like the bits and the pieces of a hologram, each and every one of us is a complete, miniature whole. Somehow, we have lost sight of the identity that defines us as minute appendages of the same tree of life that sustains all.

We are all actors and actresses in this temporary soap opera we call life. If we truly represent the embodiment of the "whole in part," then we are all gods, camouflaged in the garb of individuality, completely oblivious to the knowledge that can set us free from this grand illusion we call life.

Throughout the millennia, mystics, prophets, and philosophers have tried to share this knowledge in simple folk language time after time. Like a black hole, however, the maya of individuality, which in truth cloaks the face of reality, veils the light of our vision by continually sucking us into the center of that captivating drama, that endeared game we call "the human life."

The burden therefore is on us to wake up and free ourselves from our illusory dreams. If we truly knew that we are all but *one*, we would not fight, there would be no wars, and violence would simply not exist. We would not inflict pain on others, because we would know that by doing so, we would literally hurt ourselves. We would know that our actions have a direct impact on everything that exists.

THE WONDERS OF NATURE

In an ever-evolving effort to express itself, nature smothers the face of our planet with an unimaginable gift of plenitude. Behind me, before me, above me, or below me, I see candid hints of immeasurable profusion and amplitude. Everywhere I look, every direction high or low, I see a miraculous blossom of riches that lies beyond my field of vision, beyond the boundaries that I can humanly go. How can anyone possibly account for such prosperity, for such abundance, for such overflow?

The grains of sand, the blades of grass, the trees in the forests, the drops of rain, the blue skies, and the vastness of the infinite space all testify to the surplus and the overabundance of the endless gifts that surround me in all directions. Wherever I go, a limitless source of abundance seems to follow me with an inwardly inconceivable consistency. Everywhere I look, I see obvious signs of redundancy cradled in its infancy.

The wasteful supply of oxygen, nitrogen, carbon, and other vital components that sustain life permeate the world around me. They make up the air I breathe, the water I drink, and the very food I eat. In fact, my body is made out of the same stuff I breathe, drink, and eat. Everywhere I look, I find evidence of abundance, overproduction, excess, and overflow. In fact, I am literally submerged in a sea of expansive exuberance that incidentally fills the world.

The deep ocean beds host a mind-numbing array of

marine life. Billions of solar bodies illuminate the night skies with a feast of flickering lights. The radiant golden beams of the sun shower my body with a spectacular display of shimmering photon rays of light. They effortlessly charge me with vital energy and force of life. Who is all this copious abundance created for?

This is my abode, my turf, my bounty, the jurisdiction of my dominion, and absolute sovereignty. This planet with all its treasured belongings is a mere playground, created solely for me to develop, unfold, and harness my latent powers and faculties.

This planet is a virtual deck, uniquely erected to help me express myself. It is assembled to help me realize my true nature and to ultimately discover my inner self. We are all wizards; we are all gods and goddesses, luxuriously roaming about on the surface of this magnificent planet, experiencing the drama of physical life.

Alas, we have forgotten the memory of this divine heirship. Instead, we see ourselves as mere feeble mortals, helplessly enslaved in bondage, at the mercy of the trials and the tribulations that rise out of the circumstances.

Somehow, we find ourselves surrounded by conditions that seem to be hopelessly beyond our control. If we just distanced ourselves from our situations for a moment, however, we would easily see how, like infants lying in the cradle, we are utterly smothered with abundance, devotion, and love in a motherly tone.

Don't you see? All the greatest gifts and all the fundamental and essential constituents of life are readily at our disposal, without any intentional effort on our part to make them ours. We don't oversee the intricate operation and function of our vital organs; we don't actively try to repair our damaged cells; we don't consciously gasp for air. We don't have to do anything to watch our bodies grow; we don't need to deliberately do anything to breathe or make our hair grow. We just leave things alone and let nature direct the flow.

We are literally surrounded with an endless supply of wondrous gifts. We are blindly flooded with an overwhelming bounty that just persists. It's amazing how in the midst of all this unsparing excess, with all the multitudinous arrangements of planets, moons, stars, and solar systems, with all the galaxies and the mass firmament in celestial heavens, many of us still think that nature is deficient when it comes to life's most fundamental needs for wealth, comfort, beauty, and health.

Without a doubt, we have an infinitely abundant supply of all the elemental ingredients needed to bloom and grow in life. We have a right, not only to be alive but to flourish and thrive. Beginning with that first breath, our birth cries are comforted with an unlimited supply of air, water, sunshine, joy, love, laughter, health, happiness, and wealth.

Somehow, however, somewhere along the way, we get bored and forget to appreciate the magic of life. We somehow begin to accept lack and limitation as what is presumed to be par for the course in our journeys on the highway of life.

As we reach adulthood, we strive to conform to the norm; we subconsciously adopt habits and beliefs that tend to veil the true image of this abundant life. We slowly close the floodgates that allow the free flow of the unbounded gifts we once so unpretentiously enjoyed in life.

Gifts like air, water, food, and light are impossible to overlook, because they are needed for and fundamental in sustaining life. Others, however, like love, joy, wealth, and happiness, do not seem so crucial and can therefore be easily ignored throughout life. Though often neglected, these decidedly unnecessary gifts still endlessly remain at our disposal.

When acknowledged, they can help greatly reinforce, augment, and, if anything, adorn the tree of life. They are eternally present, lying intimately coiled up in our hearts. They remain idle, waiting to be reclaimed, waiting for us to rediscover them as we ride through the winding journey of life.

We *can* reclaim them; we can redeem them if we but have a sincere desire to once again reaffirm them in our hearts. Before we can once again reclaim these gifts, however, we would have to realize them in our imaginations and include them in our private daily monologues.

THE RAYS OF CHANGE

The rays of change are lighting up the horizon. At last, the illusion of individuality, which cloaks the fundamental nature of reality, is beginning to give way to a candid wave of transparent solidarity. We are learning to finally understand that the personal world we consciously hear, touch, smell, taste, and see may not necessarily represent the universal nature of reality. We are finally learning that our five senses may be providing a distorted or incomplete picture of reality.

This new era of information and technology, backed by quantum jargon and scientific terminology, is little by little dissolving our false sensory impressions of material solidity. Although the presumed solid object we irrefutably see with our eyes or hold and touch with our hands may seem like a lifeless mass, it is in reality a natural, living thing.

Indiscernible to the casual eye, this solid thing is made out of molecules, atoms, electrons, and other primordial elements, resonating at dizzying speeds. It affects people, places, and things through nature's invisible forces like gravity, radiation, and magnetic fields. On a cosmic scale, this whole universe we call home is a living organism, an orderly life form, composed of an inconceivable number of living parts and pieces that collectively help create the reality we all take part in.

Left on our own, out in the cold, without a guiding hand, seemingly helpless and all alone, we humans find ourselves hopelessly lost in a blinding storm. It seems we are completely oblivious to the central role we all play in this dynamic world. It's time we became aware of the crucial role we all play in the creation of this cosmic bowl.

We are beginning to understand that we are communal pieces and parts of a collective whole. We are at last beginning to see that our dissimilarities in reality represent the different colors of a universal rainbow.

We are witnessing a mind revolution that is changing the landscape of science, language, and culture in practically every organized nation on Earth. We are undergoing a transformation that is redefining the way we approach knowledge—call it a new beginning, call it a rebirth. Time has come to bid farewell to the fragmented ways of the old. It's time to embrace the new cohesive order that promises to enlighten the hearts of the weary and the minds of the old.

Science is finally giving us a glimpse of that infinite power, which awaits us when we put our minds to work and utilize our inherent faculties to advance life for everyone as a whole. People all around the world are slowly reconciling their differences and familiarizing themselves with the concept of a united Earth.

The fate of humanity as a whole is headed toward a collective state of enlightenment, a process of renaissance, a means of rebirth that is sweeping the world. We are after all beginning to understand our individual, interactive roles as the masterminds behind the wonderful drama we play in this magical world.

We are all gods; we humans are sleeping giants. Alas,

we are forgetful; we are endowed with amnesic minds. Somehow through the process of birth, we have lost the memories that link us to our divine heirship, to our right and title to rule the world. We are slowly awakening, however, and reclaiming our thrones. We are doing it by finally believing in ourselves, by believing in the collective power of our creative minds.

It's the power of imagination you know that's responsible for all the recent advancements we have witnessed in the history of this world. Electricity, space travel, wireless technologies, artificial intelligence, and subatomic discoveries lend only a glimpse of the power we have yet to discover in the uncharted virgin territories of this fertile world. The Internet has brought us closer together by helping us reflect on the connection we all share in this world.

We are about to open the floodgates of knowledge as we learn to share our resources and build equitable venues to reach our ideal goals. Our lives are so much easier than those of our predecessors, because we have learned to put our minds together and collectively grow. Scientists tell us that we use only a small portion of our mental faculties at best, but they fail to give us the blueprint with which we can engage the rest.

The wheel of evolution, however, is automatically calculating our trajectory as we delve deep into the heart of scientific mystery. Just imagine: our technological advances so far are but a drop in the bucket when we think of what the future may hold. Inherent in this realization, there is an inexpressible sense of liberation, an indescribable feeling of happiness and joy.

The greatest catalyst of human advancement and growth is to have the opportunity to realize the ultimate connection one shares with humanity, with the universe, with the cosmos in whole. The greatest contribution one can make in the name of human development and collective growth is to realize one's role as an individual unit that can make or break the orderly growth and the harmony of the whole. Don't you see it? We are all swimming in the same fishbowl. We are all just bits and pieces of one big symphony, one collective whole.

We literally share everything; we exchange the same air, the same molecules, and the same atoms that circulate around the world. We are all basically made out of the same recycled world. Life just simply becomes easier when we as individuals can collectively learn to share our resources, our talents, our experiences, our stories, and our goals.

It becomes so much better when each individual can consciously learn that he or she can contribute to the world by being happy, by feeling healthy, by living with immeasurable prosperity and joy. After all, aren't these what we are all looking for? That is exactly what this book is for.

CHAPTER 2

The Riddle of Disease and Illness

It's difficult to be productive when you are physically ill, isn't it? Being sick makes it hard to stay consistently effective, doesn't it? Disease is like an earthquake; it distracts you, shakes your foundation, sucks your energy, and saps the fresh essence of life out of you.

When you feel unwell, your outlook on life takes a different spin. Life as you know it slows down, your work and family suffer; everything gets placed on hold.

When you are ill, your energy dwindles, your sense of imagination becomes clouded, your spirit of giving loses steam, and your sense of adventure becomes a dim projection on a dark movie screen. In effect, your aspirations for success, happiness, and prosperity become foolish reveries you once held in a distant dream.

The principle is simple: health is essential for optimal productivity, a must for proper mental activity, a prerequisite for emotional stability. You need to feel healthy to be creative; you need to be at your best to feel innovative. You have to be healthy to feel romantic; you need to feel well to be artistic.

When you feel well, you are more likely to be successful in completing the job at hand, you are more inclined to extend a helping hand; you tend to be better equipped to grow and understand. In health, you seem to find more time to love others and serve them firsthand.

So what can you do to keep a healthy card on hand? Even with all the recent medical advancements, with all the health-related research, technology, and science, we are still clueless about the inner workings of this mass of meat, skin, and bones we ignorantly embody.

We've had the same body for thousands of years, and yet we are unable to cure it of even a fraction of the illnesses to which it is heir. Of all the countless concoctions, remedies, and medications we have discovered or engineered so far, none can cure even the common cold. We just do not understand the subtle secrets our bodies naturally hold. Can anyone tell me why we get sick and become old?

MIND-BODY DYNAMICS

Our bodies are made up of tissues, organs, and systems that work in harmony to carry out the function of life. These tissues and organs are made out of cells that, among other things, help form the body, communicate, produce energy, and sustain life.

When in tune with one another, every cell, every tissue, and every organ works in unison to help support the gift of life. What's important to realize, however, is that life itself is not generated by cells or any of the physical constituents of life. These are mere vehicles that are used to support the activity of physical life.

Though the body is composed of these finer living constituents, without a conscious mind, it has no intelligence to sustain life. For this reason, the condition of the body can never be separated from the mind. Therefore, a healthy body must by default reside in a healthy mind.

Moreover, the mind and body need a stream of consciousness to help generate the spark and support the function of life. Ultimately, the stream of consciousness that animates the mind and body is your higher self.

According to science, the cells in the body are renewed at least once every few months. If so, who then is it that maintains this shape and form we call ours? Who else but the higher self?

Picture this: what happens when someone dies? As soon as the mind withdraws, the body begins to decay and decompose rapidly before our eyes. The organs become lifeless, the cells burst or shrivel, and the whole body becomes a playground for other live organisms that feed on those parts. This process makes it possible to recycle the waste and eventually recapture the essential elements needed to create new lives.

What then keeps the body intact before someone dies? What is it that immunizes it from outside harm? This integrative force is none other than that essence of nature called the higher self. This higher self is an indivisible part of a universal consciousness.

So where in the body can you possibly find this higher self? So far, the answer to this question is one that no one has been able to shelf. This conscious higher self is the source that gives life to the mind itself.

The brain is said to be the seat of the consciousness. This may be true, but can anyone argue that the cells and the organs elsewhere in the body are completely devoid of this consciousness?

Every single living cell in the body is endowed with a wonderful intelligence that is intimately supported by this higher consciousness. Consciousness therefore is not limited or confined to the brain; the whole body is adorned with a matrix that accommodates this consciousness.

Our cells therefore are not just isolated, self-serving cells; they are intelligent little beings that work in harmony with one another to consciously help nourish and protect our bodies and keep them well. Together, they form an intricate communication grid that is embodied by this consciousness.

As such, they are delicate little conscious beings that can react not only to physical injuries or microscopic invasions but also to the sentiments we inadvertently entertain in our minds. These sentiments are incidentally shaped by our internal images, emotions, and inner thoughts.

Our cells have the capacity to dynamically eavesdrop on our internal emotions and monologues. In fact, they not only eavesdrop but also collectively react to the context of our emotions and mental states overall.

The nature and the extent of these reactions of course vary considerably among individuals. Depending on the circumstances, our cells can release a whole host of healing or toxic substances, which may inadvertently unfold conditions that we would not otherwise consciously intend at all.

As a matter of fact, each cell is able to change its own internal programming in response to our emotions and thoughts. In times of stress, it can communicate with other cells and send out signals to self-destruct.

Indeed, based on this perspective, one can easily argue that many of the common chronic conditions or even some cancers may be linked to our deeply embedded sentiments, emotions, or deranged patterns of thought. Many of these conditions can be potentially traced back to a long-term grudge, a source of resentment, a story of greed or anger that the individual has long held captive deep in the secret chambers of his or her heart.

Our bodies are essentially plastic: they conform to the quality of our thoughts. We literally reshape and re-form our bodies daily according to the quality of our emotions and thoughts.

We express ourselves with the bodies we assemble through the images we hold in our thoughts. We are constantly creating, maintaining, and destroying our cells by subconsciously objectifying our emotions and thoughts within the physical matrix of our minds.

MIND OVER BODY

The influence of mind over the body has been well acknowledged since the ancient years. Even in this modern era, physicians have been referring patients with chronic or acute physical conditions to psychologists and psychiatrists for years.

Mental training and psychological conditioning often treat physical conditions that have failed medical therapy for long years. Mental coaching has been known to aid in the process of health and healing for years.

It has now been scientifically proven that many disorders and conditions are best treated when the treatment plan includes behavioral guidance and positive reinforcements. This is why often patients recovering from traumatic injuries undergo a rigorous regimen of physical and occupational therapies that are highlighted by positive reinforcement and active encouragement.

The concept of mind over matter is not by any means new. In times of need, the human mind has been known to defy the tenets of rationality from every view. Look around you: how else can you explain the living examples of miraculous recovery, though they may be scattered and few?

People go without getting sick for years. Many can manage to postpone the onset of symptoms from an illness year after year. Important goals and milestones can push back this onset for an untold number of years. A child's first dance, his first recital, or her first championship game may all be important enough for a parent to remain strong and disease free for years.

Once-in-a-lifetime occasions like trips, weddings, and graduations can greatly influence our tolerance, immunity, and susceptibility to disease and pain. The common flu, for example, can wait for you to finish your exam, come back from a vacation, or get done with your audition.

The colossal potential of the human mind is a monumental force that, when called upon, can defy the laws of nature or even cheat death. We have all either lived with, read of, or been told the tale of those exceptional caregivers, overworked mothers, or otherwise busy people who openly confess they "have no time to get sick." Could it be possible for the human mind to bend the rules or change the limits of reality this way?

The truth is that the thoughts and the emotions we constantly entertain in our minds determine how our bodies function and ultimately behave in our lives. Our thoughts and emotions ultimately dictate the quality of our lives.

Favorable or not, psychological moods, factors, and variables can produce physical effects by causing chemical changes in our cells. Bad news, for example, can give you an upset stomach. Depending on its nature or severity, it may even damage your gastrointestinal cells.

Severe stress can actually alter one's physiology or even damage the body's vital cells. It can be forceful enough to trigger inflammatory reactions or even serious ulcers. It has the potential to create aging spells or even disease monsters. Deeply rooted fear, anger, or anxiety can permanently change our postures.

Anger can alter the breathing pattern and affect the process of digestion. Fear can make you quiver, feel cold, or look pale. When you are scared, your pupils dilate, your knees begin to feel weak, and a number of your bodily secretions come to a halt.

Anxious thoughts can alter the blood pressure or change the heart rate. They can cause headache, nausea, vomiting, or other similar symptoms that at least on the surface may remain unexplained.

Your mental status has the potential to deteriorate your health. It can also rejuvenate your body and help it breathe with new life. Your mind can trigger sexual arousal, cause inflammation, or help circulate a whole host of internal analgesics with calming effects.

Your mental states have the potential to induce significant physiologic effects. They have the power to trigger unnecessary immune reactions. They can instigate an untold number of positive or negative systemic reactions.

Your mind has the power to trigger neurosecretions that bring joy to your heart. Joyful news can bring tears to your eyes. Expression of love can make you blush or give you the "butterflies."

Your mind can potentially solicit a far-reaching physiologic response. It has the power to compromise your health by virtue of unresolved scars. It has a keen ability to rev up the body's stress response.

In time, this stress response can trigger the release of

various toxic substances, which may altogether damage the cells' functional or structural parts. It may lead to mutations, which are often harmless but have the potential to cause significant harm.

These are only a few examples where our minds can exert a seemingly short-term physiologic response. Unfortunately, the consequences that may follow are not necessarily always apparent all at once. In many instances, their effects run much deeper and last much longer than they seem to appear all at once.

Damaged cells in general may have an impaired ability to reproduce, maintain, protect, or repair their own parts. They may eventually make our bodies susceptible to organ damage or tissue compromise. They can induce a whole host of chronic or life-threatening conditions or just adversely affect health otherwise.

In the end, all these effects are mediated by the stimulation of nerves, the secretion of glands, and the release of substances around our cells. But these are all effects; ultimately, it's the mind that's responsible for all these effects.

Everyone knows that good hygiene, healthy foods, and plenty of sleep help, but these are not by any means sufficient enough to ensure a healthy and vibrant life. If your ailment is a by-product of your negative mental attitudes and patterns in life, could these interventions be comprehensive enough to help you live a healthy life?

Vitamins, minerals, potions, nostrums, and healing plants have existed in one form or another from the beginning of time. Despite an everlasting, unquenchable propensity for popularity, however, on their own, they seem to have no significant influence on consistently averting the threat of disease in anyone's life.

Fresh air, clean water, sunshine, conscious food consumption, and moderate physical exercise, though essential, paint only a partial picture of the ingredients needed to prevent disease and promote a healthy life. Medicines and other natural remedies are often temporary measures that at best mask the symptoms but rarely have the curative power that is so often needed in life. That's why you need to take them regularly if you wish to maintain a reasonable quality of life.

Indifferent to this crucial concept, many doctors, surgeons, practitioners, and healers, with all their books, tools, scientific machines, and magical techniques still feel helpless when they themselves succumb to disease and come down with ailments. In light of all this, isn't it easy to see how diet, exercise, and even medicine combined are practically powerless when you ignorantly suffer from a chaotic, negative, or unruly state of mind?

Don't you see that *you* are indeed orchestrating all these spells? Considering this, isn't it easy to see how many of the unexplained or chronic ailments people suffer from can be traced back to their negative or unruly states of mind?

To have a disease-free body, you need to train yourself to maintain a balanced state of mind. You need to flush your harmful mental states and reprogram your mind. You need to remove the negative mental obstacles you challenge yourself with day in and day out. You need to purge the undesirable mental and emotional states you recklessly erect for yourself month in and month out. Therefore, needless to say, the first thing you should always examine in the name of health and healing is that which takes root from the inside out.

Balanced emotions and healthy thoughts sew the fertile seeds for healthy starts. Healthy living is a by-product of healthy thoughts. Therefore, the most important part of anyone's diet should be a regimen of healthy thoughts.

Notice the word regimen, because, though essential, random healthy thoughts have no power to affect anything at all. A wavering mind has no power to heal the body at all. The key to success in this endeavor is consistency; nothing else can affect your health as much as this.

In this game then, the best strategy is to adopt a powerful daily routine that supports a healthy mind. This form of daily mental training revitalizes your body, renews your senses, and lays a firm foundation for you to maintain a healthy and vibrant life.

THE MYSTERIOUS ALCHEMY

When, in the passage of time, races forget to perceive the deeper, underlying realities that exist, the more subtle substratum of life, where the true powers of the individual lie, gets buried and becomes obscured, as if by an esoteric mist. The hypnotizing effects of this obscuring mist blinds people to the unlimited potential powers they can possibly enlist. As a result, the more superficial aspects of life take precedence, leaving limited resources for individuals to consciously will or to consciously create.

Throughout history, sages and scholars have time and again tried to remove this mist. The illusion of the physical world, however, continues to cloak the true nature of the deeper levels that invariably exist. Whether we are aware of it or not, these subtle levels still exist. The only difference is that we recklessly dabble in them without ever really knowing the consequences they can potentially enlist.

By nature, thoughts have the power to operate both in the grosser as well as these subtler realms. Essentially, on one level, we can see the direct effect of thought on the body by observing some of the brain's voluntary commands. For example, many of our muscles are under the control of the will. That's how we can speak and move our limbs. In these settings, a mere thought causes the brain to send signals through the nerves and affect distant muscles or target organs.

What many of us fail to see, however, is that our

thoughts may also have a pronounced subconscious effect on the welfare of our individual cells. This may not be necessarily mediated through direct connections or individual nerves. Here, the mind may work in subtler ways.

For instance, your subconscious thoughts or emotions may ultimately determine how lifeless or healthy you look and feel inside. Since the mind and the body are intimately intertwined, the thoughts that penetrate the barriers of your subconscious mind eventually build the foundation on which your physical body is enshrined. A healthy body therefore is by default embalmed in a healthy mind.

The greatest work of alchemy we all engage in throughout life is the unconscious way we turn our thoughts and emotions into the physical molds we inadvertently embody in life. Once you understand the delicate nature of this biological alchemy, you should be able to realize your potential in achieving and maintaining a life that is essentially disease free. You should be able to use this knowledge to transmute and transform your current body into one that is an unfailing source of health, energy, and vitality.

This way, you are better able to reach the positive outcomes you wish to experience in life. The pages that follow reveal the apparent but seemingly inconsequential trivialities that in fact immensely impact one's reality. Learn them well, because having a keen understanding of these fundamentals will have a tremendous bearing on how you influence your quality of life and state of health.

THE ROLE OF THOUGHT

Like light particles that tirelessly float and seamlessly collide, literally trillions and trillions of thoughts flash in and out of the back screen of the wondering mind. They effortlessly flow in rhythmic waves, thrashing about, seeking attention, fading in and out of consciousness.

We churn out thoughts as if they are produced by exceptionally efficient machines. Whether we are aware of it or not, we literally entertain thousands and thousands of thoughts from the time we wake up until the moment we fall asleep.

It doesn't stop there, however; we continue to form thoughts even as we enter the deeper stages of dream and sleep. Like a television station, we receive, generate, and broadcast thoughts, which are often visual and in random streams.

We are relentlessly driven to constantly think. We think as we read, as we drive, or as we brush our teeth. We think as we comb our hair or even as we subconsciously breathe. We think as we work, eat, talk, or even listen to the radio or watch TV.

A great majority of these thoughts clutter the mind. Some grab our attention, while eventually a handful help shape our destinies. All in all, however, the most perplexing part of it all is that the majority of what we normally think about is a mixed bag of random, pointless thoughts that never really helps us accomplish anything.

The point I am trying to make here is that we have the

power to control our streams of thought. We have the power to take advantage of them to help us connect our lives' most important dots. Why are thoughts suddenly so important you ask?

Most people inherently believe that thoughts are inconsequential. They think that a thought is by description an ethereal, fluffy mental construct that has no true bearing on the nature of reality at all, but in fact it does. Thoughts form the fundamental basis of what creates reality. They are in essence quantum, nonmaterial units of energy and information that have an intrinsic effect on the nature of this physical reality.

Thoughts carry the monumental force against which this whole universe seems to be powerless. They are impregnated with a force that stems from the core of causality, the same force that directs the creation of all things. We are in fact the creators of that force; we generate that force and then disseminate it in the form of thought.

In a way, a thought is a tool with which we can express the mysterious, ethereal projections of our creative minds. Inherent in this expression, there is energy and information, which get naturally transformed and translated into the solid realities we perceive with our senses and with our minds.

Thoughts weave the fabric of the realities we experience in our lives. Incidentally, the intensity and the awareness with which we emanate them into space may actually determine the speed with which they promptly manifest.

Regardless of speed, however, in every case our

thoughts inevitably get incorporated into the seemingly solid realities we perceive with our senses and our minds. If this is not so readily apparent, it's because we are distracted and forgetful; we just can't seem to connect the dots. We forget that we are the actual bearers of the cause.

You see, the lag time between the generation of a thought and its materialization may sometimes take days, weeks, months, or even eons. In order to materialize, a thought may sometimes have to travel from here all the way to Mars. In other words, the materialization of the substance of our thoughts may oftentimes be preceded by a long, pregnant pause.

Even though we create our own individual realities through our thoughts, we live in a world community where reality is being created by collective thoughts. In spite of all this, each and every one of us sees a subtle version of reality that is slightly different, one that supports his or her own subtle presumptions, perceptions, and individual thoughts.

We are all therefore literally creating our own individual realities through our thoughts. This should shed light on why some people are generally happy, while others seem to always suffer without an apparent cause. It should explain why some people wallow in poverty, while others are drowned in wealth, feeling insulated from the harsh realities others seem to always materialize.

Look around yourself; everything you work with, everything you see around you is a product of thought. Just about everyone agrees that all the human-made objects in this world are the products of thought. Interestingly enough, very few can see the intimate connection between their thoughts and the physical realities they actually construct.

The quality of your thoughts clothe you in the form of flesh. They define your characteristic behaviors and determine the nature of your interactions with others. Can you not see it?

Thoughts can make or break you; they can mandate health, happiness, wealth, poverty, or sickness. Even your physical appeal, your charisma, your magnetic presence, and your dominating beauty or crudeness are all the products of nothing but mere thoughts.

You are the master builder; you are the architect and the designer of your life. Your thoughts are the brick and mortar with which you erect the frame that literally molds your body, your circumstances, and ultimately your entire life.

Thoughts carry enough potential to alter the course of not only your life but the whole multidimensional universe, the very playground that is spun in the cobweb of life. Thoughts have gravitational and repulsive forces that indeed extend far beyond the imagination of an average individual mind.

Consciously or not, through thoughts you form your own preferences, rituals, or addictions. Through thoughts you form the propensities with which you inadvertently assemble your circles of enemies and friends. The quality of your thoughts predisposes you to the nature of the jobs you choose, the partners you pick, and the friends you attract.

Through thoughts, you literally attract the squalor and the wretchedness, or the luxury and the happiness you surround yourself with in life. Your health and vitality, your physical challenges, your sickness and decrepitude, your subjective age or state of youth are nothing but the by-products of your thoughts in truth.

Thoughts represent the vibrational expressions of the mind's creative force. Using the brain, the endocrine, and the nervous systems, these vibrations act on atoms and molecules to mold the body we subconsciously create in our lives. Therefore, the condition of the body depends on the quality of not only the brain, the endocrine, or the nervous systems, but more importantly our thoughts.

Thoughts are like wireless signals that invisibly surround us. They zip in and out of our bodies and infiltrate the world around us. They penetrate solid objects and permeate distances far beyond us.

In general, we not only generate thoughts but also have an affinity for thought vibrations that closely match ours. We readily absorb and act on those that conform to the habits and the interests that are more closely in line with ours. If we feel stressed or down all the time, we will continue to attract thoughts that resonate with and ultimately strengthen that state of mind.

Literally, every cell in the body is conscious of its state of mind. Those that are nourished by a healthy state of mind create bodies that are strong, balanced, and ultimately refined. On the other hand, those that are constantly threatened by unhealthy, sickly, negative, or distorted thoughts are destined to identify themselves with bodies that are weak, sedentary, corruptible, and prone to illness all the time.

Knowing all this, wouldn't it be prudent to plan ways and means of controlling the thoughts you entertain in your life? Learn to become conscious of the fact that your thoughts can dictate your state of health and the direction you head toward in life. Learn to become aware of the nature of your thoughts. Learn to realize the influence they may have in creating and maintaining a healthy life.

What kind of thoughts would you say you normally entertain in your daily life? Do you feel overworked? Are you depressed? Are you constantly worried about some unforeseen health-related situation or circumstance? Are you anxious all the time? Do you feel sickly and tired all the time? Are you suffering from aches and pains that seem to wax and wane all the time?

Learn to identify the habitual thoughts that keep you mesmerized with your unhealthy patterns in life. Learn to replace those that get in your way and prevent you from experiencing a healthy life. There is nothing quite so healing or invigorating as thoughts that help promote and create a healthy and vibrant life.

Revitalize yourself; generate thoughts that resonate to the tune of a healthy and vibrant life. Raise your internal vibrations with thoughts that gravitate around peace, harmony, beauty, health, joy, healing, and love.

Be patient; the results you would expect to see from these thoughts do not normally tend to surface overnight. Ordinarily, the body responds little by little, not overnight. That's why a drastic cure or change is unlikely until you immerse your mind in them for a considerable amount of time.

With practice, eventually we can all create the pliability and the flexibility needed to generate and maintain a body that is ultimately healthy and physically fit for life. Keep reading to learn how to replace your negative thoughts with those that can actually help you cultivate and experience a healthy life.

THE ROLE OF EMOTIONS

In a naive and simplistic way, emotions can be thought of as physiological markers that are triggered by mere thoughts. They refer to a state of consciousness where both the mind and the body are involved in expressing a thought.

Perhaps thoughts and emotions are inseparable expressions of a thinking animal or human mind. Conceivably, emotions can be said to signify the intensity of a streaming thought. A sudden change in behavior or an intense outward expression are often telltale signs that emotions may be strongly involved.

Common physical findings when emotions are aroused may include tears in the eyes, flushing of the skin, wrinkles on the forehead, laughter, or changes in tone, speech, or posture. As such, many of our emotions like anger, fear, happiness, sadness, lust, and love may in general visibly manifest themselves in different organs or body parts.

Therefore, our emotions are selectively interwoven into the functional fabric of practically every organ and every body part. Some of them are so powerful, they can alter the mental status, affect homeostasis, or influence the processes of digestion, secretion, or excretion.

Essentially, emotions may in a way represent thoughts that are hyperlinked to the body's autonomic response. In this framework, they are mere thoughts that are endogenously associated with a physiologic response. Fear, for example, is a perception that may result in loss of appetite.

It may dilate the eyes, halt digestion, increase the heart rate, or trigger a fight-or-flight response.

Certain emotions may activate the salivary glands or trigger a hunger response. Sexual arousal may provoke a complex interplay of influences that often involve a multisystemic response. Grief can cause a whole host of disturbances that may precipitate a serious endogenous response.

Of course, some emotions are regulatory and vital. They form some of the most primitive instincts and visceral impulses that are necessary for survival. Some are so hardwired, they are easily able to bypass the orderly, conscious, decision-making processes of the reasoning human mind. In short, some emotions can easily override and dictate one's state of health and well-being in life.

At birth, it seems, we come preprogrammed with a set of rudimentary emotions that undeniably serve to help us survive. Ideally, however, as we grow older, we begin to learn ways to consciously understand, use, and better manage our emotions in life. In this process, we are in effect striving to become more civilized and socially wiser in life.

If we don't, we will continue to helplessly react to the surge of feelings that constantly serve to undermine our inherent physical or psychological states in life. In this mind-set, we are at best leading a crude, animalistic form of life.

Strong feelings and intense emotions, if left unchecked, can often adversely affect health and deteriorate the quality of life. As a general rule, though essential for survival, if left untamed, primitive emotions may not necessarily be conducive to shaping or supporting a healthy life.

Emotions in general can be intense, irrational, and potentially self-destructive. When uncontrolled, they have the power to adversely direct the course of our lives. Unfortunately, we don't understand the intricate role they play in influencing the decisions we make or the actions we take in our day-to-day lives. When dictated by emotions, our decisions and actions keep creating stressful situations that tend to color the quality of our daily lives.

When negative emotions like fear, anger, hatred, jealousy, and distrust take root and become persistent, they gain enough power to trigger an endogenously toxic stress response. The repercussions that may follow can ultimately affect the physiology or cause significant harm. When these emotions run rampant for decades, day after day and month after month, they can silently change the constitution of the body and make it ultimately underperform.

Therefore, to promote and maintain a healthy lifestyle, it is essential to control the way our emotions inherently influence our lives. In the end, it's the initiative and the knowledge of controlling our emotions that sets us apart from other animals that populate the lower forms of life.

The idea of controlling our emotions here does not imply a radical form of sensory denial. On the contrary, it's a means of gaining mastery over our primitive, impulsive urges that incidentally control what we say, think, or do in life. By gaining mastery over the triggers that push our emotional buttons, we can learn to live a healthier and more balanced life.

THE UNDERLYING CAUSES

Why do we get sick? This is but one of the many unanswered questions that have plagued the mind of humanity since the beginning of time. The moment modern science finds a way to eradicate something, a newer, more complex mechanism of disease emerges just to complicate things.

We study disease from a variety of angles, including bacteriology, virology, physiology, biochemistry, and genetics to name only a few. What we mysteriously fail to see, however, is that these mechanisms do not describe the underlying cause; they just simply provide clues.

Have you ever wondered why in a percentage of those who are clinically cured, the disease may return in only a matter of days, weeks, or months? In such cases, although the signs and the symptoms of the disease may be provisionally gone, is it possible that perhaps the underlying cause, the source of infliction, may have otherwise remained fundamentally strong?

Have you ever wondered why identical twins in the same household, under the same conditions, may respond differently to the same disease or supposed cause? Why is it that while one may be diagnosed with a genetic disease, the other may not be affected at all? How do you explain why from time to time, health-care professionals may unknowingly work around highly infectious individuals, without coming down with a serious disease at all?

Is it possible to imagine that when it comes to disease, the primary source or cause may rest outside the scope of physical laws? Is it possible to argue that genetic, metabolic, or infectious diseases by themselves can never be the primary source or cause? Perhaps we are too engrossed in the physical body to acknowledge that the source may altogether rest on what constitutes a nonphysical cause.

This is not a novel idea; philosophers, psychologists, psychiatrists, and even quantum scientists have long analyzed the concept of causality, debating the degree of influence of mind over physical reality. In fact, in the quantum world, the wave of potentiality does not collapse into physical reality without the mind entering into it.

In other words, it's the mind that solidifies what the individual interprets as physical reality. Could the human mind in actuality be the main perpetrator behind disease, morbidity, and mortality?

Simply said, the non-Newtonian science, the new science of this century, implies that mere attention or observation can in essence create reality. In other words, even though there is a general consensus about what describes reality, each and every one of us sees a subtle version of reality that is slightly different, one that supports his or her own subtle presumptions, perceptions and concepts of individual reality.

This means that each and every one of us literally crystalizes an individual glimpse of reality from an infinite selection of possibilities. Therefore, consciously or not, by focusing on things that cause discomfort and disease, we can actually manifest the physical characteristics that are in line with those realities. Naturally, the reverse can also hold true.

FALLEN DREAMS

When it comes to understanding our bodies, the first thing we must realize is that we are spiritual beings, not physical machines. Our physical bodies are vehicles we have unconsciously adopted to express ourselves within the natural order of things. Like the snake that periodically sheds its skin, science tells us that every so often, we replace nearly every cell in the body, as if we are creating new vehicles for ourselves to operate in.

In childhood, we tend to constantly dream up new bodies that help us grow taller, stronger, healthier, and more fit. As we get older, however, we forget to dream up new dreams. We forget to create new bodies and therefore naturally fall prey to old age and degenerative disease.

If you want to feel youthful, if you want a healthy body, you need to once again dream and think like children do. You need to keep shaping and reshaping a new body in your imagination, like children do.

In general, disease and old age begin to surface when we get bored with things, when we no longer grow with the flow of things. In childhood, we dream of adventure; we dream of growing up and doing all kinds of wonderful things. We dream of being smarter and wiser; we dream of conquering things.

These dreams in essence form a fountain of youth that we subconsciously use to restore and renew ourselves in. By dreaming up these childish dreams, we get to literally bathe our bodies in a healing spring.

Unfortunately, by the time we reach adulthood, most of us forget that we need to continue to dream. Somehow, we fail to realize that it was the nature of dreaming itself that kept us youthfully energized with health and zeal.

In youth, we feel indestructible; in truth, we feel strong and unsinkable. We purge pain and illness from our bodies as if they are readily dissolvable. Soon enough, however, as the sounds and the colors of life begin to lose their emotional intensity and mythical appeal, we tend to fall prey to the clutches of boredom; we gradually forget that we are actually living a golden dream.

By the time we reach adulthood, we all but lose that magical sense of wonder. Instead, distaste and weariness begin to take over. We somehow become cynical; we get bored with life. We mindlessly forget to appreciate the natural miracles we once perceived in life. We altogether forget that we live in a dream-breathed life.

What do you think of when you get up in the morning or when you go to bed at night? Your troubles? Your pains or illnesses? Your job? Your finances? Your children? Your relationship or lack thereof? Do these things let you spread your wings or make you happy in life? Do you ever dream of a strong, fit, or healthy life?

To be healthy, you need to have lofty dreams. You need to dream of learning, growing, and doing extraordinary things. Like children, you need to look forward to a future filled with happy things.

Whether you are a writer, a cook, a driver, or a rocket engineer, whether you are twenty years old or eighty, you need to constantly dream of creating a better and more exciting future. When you dream of a brighter future, your body will learn to stay healthy as long as it takes for you to create that future. So learn to keep on dreaming of a happier, healthier, and a more meaningful future.

Swimming against the Stream

Of course it would seem childish to propose a simplistic model to explain the basis of sickness and disease. However, while the causes may be rooted in a complex web of poorly understood factors and tendencies, solving the puzzle may not be as hard as it ordinarily seems.

Often, the secret may come down to understanding the consequences of forgetting that we live in a field of dreams. In this mind-set, we tend to forget that we don't have to force anything; we can just create what we want by allowing ourselves to once again dream. Instead, we try to impatiently swim against the mainstream, against the flow of nature, against the natural order and harmony of things.

Discomfort and disease often tend to surface when we try to force nature to quench our endless appetites and insecurities. They often find a way of crashing in every time we try to ignore the role of nature in creating effortlessly harmonious themes. They tend to emerge every time we try to immerse ourselves in self-serving, self-indulgent schemes.

That's because these endeavors are often associated with strong, negative feelings like greed, fear, doubt, jealousy, resentment, and many other similar things. Naturally, these feelings have a tendency to create internal friction, conflict, stress, pain, confusion, and many other similar themes. Much to our dismay, we don't realize the root cause of these things.

INTERNALIZING THINGS

As we ceaselessly struggle to force our desires against the natural flow of things, we begin to face a growing set of challenges that only serve to complicate things. These challenges often tend to be plagued by more setbacks, frustrations, and disappointing themes.

More often than not, these setbacks and frustrating themes eventually get internalized as painful lessons and undesirable dreams. Unfortunately, instead of letting go and learning from these lessons and mistaken dreams, we mindlessly hold on to them and treat them as intimate stories and personal themes.

Eventually, if held on to, these painful lessons and distasteful dreams end up creating self-imposed limitations, not to mention a restricted view of things. This can cause conflict, friction, and a whole host of other negative tendencies.

These negative attributes and tendencies eventually form a fertile playground for pain, illness, and chronic disease. In time, with every prick of pain and every bout of illness, we gradually distance ourselves from that vibrant life we were once accustomed to in our earlier years. Little by little, we inch farther and farther away from that ideal picture of health we so innocently took for granted in our formative years.

We eventually veer so far off track that perhaps one day we may find ourselves content to settle with a mere anemic, pain-averting existence, in a life filled with torment and utter misery. We become mere beggars in an empire we once so enthusiastically ruled over with such youthful pride and bravery.

When we constantly clothe ourselves with the pain we feel from the disappointments and the frustrations of our daily lives, our bodies begin to transmute and degenerate in front of our very eyes. This is how we pave the way for disease and aging to fasten their ghastly fangs upon our bodies and minds.

You see, our bodies are impressionable. Like raw clay, they shift and shape to conform to the subliminal ideas, pictures, and impressions we hold in our conscious and subconscious minds. They are in essence dynamically molded by the way we subconsciously perceive and interpret things in our lives.

Our bodies are in fact mindlessly contoured and gradually hammered into shape by the complex interactions and challenges that we inwardly accumulate and inadvertently internalize. In short, the way we interpret things, the lens through which we filter the world around us, dictates the way our bodies respond to the threat of disease in our lives.

In most cases, this process of internalization is so subtle, we rarely ever notice its destructive effects. We simply assume that aging and illness are routine processes that occur as a natural part and parcel of life. In reality, however, they occur as we recklessly accumulate and internalize things in the deepest recesses of our own minds.

In truth, your disease (whatever it may be) is perhaps a reflection of the growing burden that stems from your reckless dispositions, internalized conflicts, opposing values, and antagonistic beliefs. All these things often happen when you try to force results or otherwise control or manipulate things. They happen when you attempt to selfishly serve your own unbalanced needs.

Often disease surfaces when you forget to respect the natural order of things. The internalized pains and conflicts that arise from forcing or disrespecting the order and harmony of things weaken the immune system and cause ailments and conditions that are otherwise unforeseen.

Like flesh-eating bugs, internalized pains and conflicts tend to weaken the body's core building blocks. They tend to chew away and slowly melt its chemical bonds. This invariably leaves the body in an utter state of compromise.

Of course, on the surface, it may seem as if you've had no role in creating the disease you are currently experiencing. Perhaps you are a victim of a contagion or a metabolic or late-onset genetic condition. Maybe you are suffering from a viral or a bacterial invasion. Perchance you may be experiencing a fungal, parasitic, or a rare form of infection.

Indeed, any one of these may be true. When you think about it, however, it would be fairly easy to see that if your body is not in any way compromised, none of these can seriously affect you. Even the effect of the metabolic or genetic condition is ultimately dictated by you.

Otherwise, they should surely reproduce the same condition in those around you that have the same predisposition. This is why it's so hard to explain why others in your household may have escaped the wrath of that same storm that afflicted you.

THE FACE OF STRESS

Science tells us that our physical bodies are vulnerable to invasion by bacteria, viruses, fungi, and other living things. Luckily, it also tells us that we live in a mutually beneficial relationship with many of these microscopic things.

Those that reside on the skin, for example, can actually help prevent infection. They may even support the natural healing process in times of repair and regeneration.

Many of these organisms naturally colonize different body parts. Some may dwell on the skin, while others may populate the sweat glands or aggregate on the hair strands. Some are indigenous to the respiratory or gastrointestinal tracts.

Some are indispensable in the immunization process. Many are known to be instrumental in developing immunity or resistance. Certain geographic locations, for example, may host bugs that may be normally harmful or otherwise fatal for visitors from foreign lands.

Ordinarily, the immune system is designed to erect barriers against these creatures and protect us from harm. When it functions properly, it keeps them from spreading uncontrollably or from causing serious physical harm.

Under certain conditions, however, when the body's natural balance gets disrupted or somehow compromised, the immune system machinery can become unstable or even altogether desensitized.

What's more concerning is that at certain thresholds, the immune system can seemingly switch sides and mount an abnormal or even a counterproductive response. This may inadvertently affect healthy cells and cause them harm.

In an ensuing immune response, our cells may release chemicals that can cause serious physiologic disruption or self-harm. At times, this assault may not only affect the invading intruders but also the host cells or organs they intend to protect from harm.

Our protective mechanisms are not always accurate and clear-cut. They may at times tear the house down to destroy a minuscule spot.

The good news is that our impaired or damaged cells get repaired or recycled in a natural process that routinely takes place in our bodies around the clock. We constantly replace our damaged, old, or worn-out cells as we remodel our bodies hour by hour, day and night. This relentless process is a miracle that is constantly at work, even when we are sound asleep at night.

What's puzzling is that if we are repairing, replacing, or recycling our defective or damaged cells relentlessly night and day, why do we still fall prey to chronic diseases and disorders anyway? What's behind all this madness? What's the missing part? Is it the weather? The environment? Bad genes? Bad luck?

Most people see the human body as a fragile, isolated organism that is laden with shortcomings and built-in weaknesses. They see it as a delicate living machine that is prone to attack by unforeseen elements and processes. Human beings, however, have survived for ages despite the ongoing threats from novel diseases.

Normally, the immune system is well equipped to meet and overcome any potential threat that may come from these bugs. Somehow, however, we still manage to fall prey to the clutches of disease, thanks to these opportunistic thugs. Can anyone tell me why?

Perhaps one explanation may be because the body's immune and regenerative processes may not be optimally efficient at all times. Under normal circumstances, the body is so resilient, it can quickly rectify the problem and move on; however, under suboptimal or compromising conditions, it may not be able to recognize the threat or compensate for too long.

The natural question is, how can the body become compromised at times? Of course, chronic underlying conditions, trauma, or toxicities from food or environment can certainly play a huge role, but what if all these have been checked and accounted for?

Perhaps *stress* may play a huge role in this type of scenario. Stress is now a well-recognized health hazard that can seriously impact the quality of life. At times, it can compromise the immune system, impair the natural host response, and create havoc in life. Stress triggers are often ubiquitous and easily found in homes, schools, workplaces, or really anywhere one normally engages in the business of life.

Given the complexities of the human life, it should come as no surprise that stress can play such an important role in our lives. Stress usually surfaces when we experience unease or when we display friction toward displeasing or disagreeable things. Often, it takes flight on the wings of conflicting, frustrating, or disappointing themes.

Think about it: how often do you mull over stressful things and situations in your life? Needless to say, some people are always bound to lead a highly stressful life.

Given the unpredictable ups and downs that seem to always find their way into our day-to-day lives, it should be reasonable to expect a certain amount of stress in life. If left unrecognized or unmanaged, stress has a tremendous potential to firmly assert itself and gain a significant stronghold in our day-to-day lives.

Like a chemical spill, stress has a peculiar propensity to spread and tarnish all the healthy regions of an unbalanced body and mind. In times of stress, your body releases stress hormones, which under normal conditions serve to mobilize your body to meet its needs and keep its functions aligned.

Under the pressure of chronic stress, however, these hormones can constantly circulate in your body, and cause either a system-wide intolerance or insufficient response. In time, this can compromise your health or weaken your immune response. It can result in chronic or life-threatening conditions, ranging from the simplest to the most complex diseases and disorders that would have been extremely unlikely otherwise.

We've all heard of sudden, stress-induced conditions following a traumatic episode or experience in life. If severe enough, asthma attacks, speech impairments, or even sudden urinary incontinence are not by any means unheard of.

Following a moderately stressful event, signs of cognitive disturbance, sensory or motor deficits, or even syncope or heart attack are not necessarily unheard of. Stress, when left unchecked, can potentially mount a strong enough punch to make us sick from the inside out.

In fact, one reason many diseases become chronic or repeatedly occur over time may be because we inadvertently create or allow ourselves to thrive on the face of stress all the time. Given the adverse impact stress may have on our lives, stress management should be a priority in everyone's mind.

A great way to ensure that the body is optimally healthy at all times is to take steps to diffuse the inevitable sources of stress at key clutch times. Among a variety of strategies, there are at least two things you can teach yourself right now to significantly decrease or diffuse the source of stress in your life.

One is to control your emotions. Here, the best strategy is to prepare yourself to identify and diffuse your stress-triggering emotions in advance. This way, when a well-known trigger presents itself, you'll have a choice to either consciously respond or to diffuse its impact on your body and mind.

The other is to learn to intuitively align yourself with the natural flow and rhythm of life. When you learn to think and act in line with the natural flow of life, you are more likely to enjoy a happier and less stressful life. This is where learning to apply and trust your instinct and intuition can become a tremendous boon in your life.

CHAPTER 3

The Age-Old Secrets of Healthy Living

A CHANGE IN PARADIGM

An old paradigm is reemerging, the crux of which argues that our aches, pains, and diseases in reality originate from the inside out. To really understand this, we need to reexamine how we actually perceive our roles as human beings within the vast fabric of this living cosmos.

The first question that may come to mind is whether we are autonomous beings or the victims of a random accident-prone universe. Is it even possible to consider that we may be the cocreators of the realities we see erected around ourselves?

Who creates our bodies? How did we appear in these fleshly living frameworks we mindlessly embody? Who is ultimately responsible for caring for this body? Are we at the mercy of an ever-changing sea of circumstances? Or do we really have the power to keep ourselves healthy or even heal ourselves?

Do we really know who is in charge here? Despite thousands of years of human history, it seems we are still struggling to solve this mystery. To an outsider, it could seem as if we may be absorbed in a deep dream or in a multimillennial reverie.

Perhaps we have fallen asleep behind the wheels in status quo. Obviously, there is lot that we do not yet know. Lost in complete ignorance, as if blindfolded, it seems we have turned on the autopilot and let our bodies run the show.

Knowing this, is it any wonder to find our bodies ravaged in disease-ridden chaos, often completely out of control? Lost in this mental fog, it's a pity that we are not consciously aware of our own intimate leadership role.

At first glance, it seems preposterous to think that we can take charge and keep ourselves healthy with a mere change in paradigm. Nevertheless, when we consider the possibilities that have emerged from the field of quantum science, this idea may not really be such a far-off stretch after all.

The confusion here often stems from mindlessly believing that our bodies are isolated, self-propelled organisms that function beyond our control. The reality, however, is that we humans are timeless, spaceless souls; we constantly shape and reshape these individualized bodies through the very thoughts, words, and deeds we entertain with every grain of brain, heart, and soul.

Believe it or not, *we* are the ones that ultimately own these bodies we call ours. Consciously or not, *we* are the ones that write the faulty life scripts we so frantically try to disown as ours. Alas, we have lost our identities and forgotten our integrative roles.

We have somehow delegated the care of these bodies to our subconscious and automated controls. The sad part is that we have forgotten the inner workings of the buttons that operate these controls.

Normally, the function of the body is for the most part carefully regulated by the subconscious mind. Untouched, this work flows like a perfectly harmonious song. Fortunately or not, however, it can also be intimately influenced by the deliberations of the conscious mind.

The truth is that the subconscious mind is often subtly influenced by our daily casual conversations and inner monologues. Its delicate controls are susceptible to the predominant thoughts and the images we normally entertain in our conscious minds.

The subconscious mind is rather naive and impressionable. It may be sensitive to any form of impressive, conscious, or semiconscious event or thought. Muddy or not, the impressions it perceives may have the potential to create subtle changes in the maintenance and the operation of our bodies, whether we want it to or not.

The subconscious mind constantly works to rebuild and maintain the body, by conforming to the thoughts and the feelings we often predominantly embody. Often, our seemingly harmless feelings and thoughts are by no means innocent at all. Some, in fact, are so powerful, they can subconsciously alter the timing and the process of aging, death, puberty, and menopause.

Thoughts have the power to potentially alter our genetic makeup. They can even create a stormy shake-up. They can essentially dictate the way our bodies respond to toxic or healing stimuli. This may explain why some people tend to heal quickly, while others always feel weak or sickly.

Most people would scoff at the idea that they may have anything to do with the inflictions they are allegedly forced to bear. I am sure no one in a right mind would enjoy experiencing self-inflicted pain.

It would seem absurd to think that we would somehow willingly submit to the venomous jaws of illness and pain. The truth, however, is that the stimulus of thought can harvest enough power to affect the way our bodies react to the threat of sickness and pain.

When recklessly dwelled on for a protracted period of time, negative thoughts can draw enough power to potentially penetrate and influence the subconscious mind. They can overwhelm the mind, arouse unruly emotions, or create all sorts of ill conditions of common or exotic kind.

Once these thoughts find a way to penetrate the subconscious mind, they can gain enough momentum to create havoc from the inside out. Somehow, once inside, they seem to have a peculiar tendency to encourage thoughts of the same kind.

Naturally, this can make you feel physically impaired or weak all the time. Of course, as you would expect, thoughts of opposite character should certainly have the propensity to produce the opposite effect.

This should actually partially explain why some people come down with symptoms as soon as a rumor spreads, while others thrive in health, regardless of what the environment threads. You see, it's not some exotic bug from a faraway land that gets you; the one that sets you up to stumble is *you*.

Great empires fall, not by the force of enemies without but by the source of weakness within. If you seek health, you should stop focusing on the creatures without. Instead, you should concentrate on reinforcing the thoughts that highlight your greatness within.

In this light, it should be easy to see that *you* are the one that sets yourself up to experience the maladies you so often complain of. You create the disease monsters you are so often unutterably weary of.

The perpetrator behind all the chronic physical afflictions in your life is no one else but *you*! In reality, you have no one else to blame for your physical mishaps and sufferings but *you*. You repeatedly sow the seeds of the bitter fruits you taste in agony and despair, not realizing that the actual instigator is *you*.

You are the main culprit, not the "Martian flu"; *you* are the perpetrator, not some enemy outside of you. *You* are the master of your own destiny. In the end, *you* are the one that can prevent these inflictions for you.

The first thing you must do to break this cycle and start anew is to realize that the responsibility for your health starts with you. You must recognize the thoughts that can potentially harm you.

In this process, you will find that you must take steps to avoid many of the thoughts that you are ordinarily accustomed to. Thoughts that generate negative feelings, like fear, greed, jealousy, hatred, or anxiety to name a few, tend to naturally invoke physical factors and conditions that can potentially harm you.

In light of all this, it should be common sense to think that you can perhaps prevent or alleviate many of your ill conditions by correcting or removing the thoughts that could potentially harm you. It has been scientifically shown that on many occasions, depression, fibromyalgia, and many other severe or unexplained symptoms can readily resolve when the individual is removed from the places or situations that serve as triggers behind them all.

Slay your demons of negative thought. Pour cold water over your fire of hatred, fear, jealousy, anxiety, and doubt. Put an end to your disordered, discordant, or inharmonious thoughts. Focus on happiness, health, and harmony as your primary foods for thought.

Changing deeply rooted thoughts, especially when they have manifested as physical ailments and other faults, may sometimes require the help of gods. Lucky for us, however, there is a simple remedy that, when faithfully adhered to, can easily dislodge those thoughts.

You see, good thoughts and bad thoughts are in fact extreme opposites of the same continuum of thought. Lucky for us, our brains cannot simultaneously entertain both extremes in the same frame of mind. By choosing to constantly dwell on the most favorable forms of thought, you can not only dislodge the bad ones but also keep all the harmful intruders out.

So change your latitude; spring into a new, healthy *you*. Replace your unhealthy thoughts with their healthy counterparts. By removing the underlying cause, like a released rubber ball, the body will soon resume its natural condition and undergo a healthy overhaul.

History shows that humans have survived pandemics, plagues, viruses, and bacteria even when the knowledge of sanitation and hygiene was all but crude. We have survived against all odds, even when the healers and the witch doctors used snake oil and chicken beaks as healing food.

As a doctor of allopathic medicine, I am convinced that the only concoction that can alleviate every chronic condition known to humankind is manufactured inside the human mind. This potion is made up of thoughts that normally tend to uplift, inspire, and nurture the human mind. Hope, gratitude, laughter, happiness, and love are some of the most priceless healing ingredients that, though vital, do not need a doctor's prescription at all.

DON'T STRESS OVER THE OUTCOME

We humans are emotional creatures that move, live, and breathe on the edge of desire. Everything we do and everything we think about are ultimately founded on the heels of desire. It seems we are primarily occupied with nothing but the business of fulfilling our desires.

Our capacity to generate a virtually endless stream of desires is just incomprehensible. In fact, our incredible thirst to churn out new desires is simply unquenchable.

Whether the desire is for a thing, car, house, child, or relationship, if the impulse is strong enough, it will move us to act from the inside out. It will hold us hostage until we see the fruit of that desire or find a way to sort it out.

For some reason, fulfilling a desire seems to create an ever deeper sense of joy in our hearts. From desire to desire, we keep tirelessly pursuing that sense of fulfillment in our hearts.

Everyone knows that it's practically impossible to obtain every single thing we ever desire. So then what happens when we are unable to quench that insatiable thirst for a gnawing desire?

In some people, the inability to fulfill a long-awaited, cherished desire may generate a sentiment of unworthiness, defeat, or demeaning failure. Naturally, these feelings have the potential to emotionally suffocate its unassuming bearer. If not sorted out, the aftermath may often leave one in a painful quagmire.

This is not by any means a theoretical picture. In fact,

this process starts in childhood and continues as one accumulates the impressionable memories of each and every unfulfilled desire. It all starts when we become attached to the outcomes we expect from an intimate desire. Our childish, impatient expectations eventually grow and flare into a consuming fire.

When you act on the force of a desire, it finds an unlimited array of outcomes before it. If you keep your composure and leave yourself open to what may transpire, chances are you'll be surprised to see the potential outcome of that desire. When you limit yourself to your narrow range of expectations, however, you may soon hit resistance, get discouraged, and hastily call for a premature cease-fire.

Naturally, when you lose hope or become impatient, troublesome feelings like worry, stress, fear, or anxiety tend to swarm the mind and easily run it over. They will promptly gather to rain on your parade and steal your thunder.

In the beginning, these feelings may affect the body by generating simple side effects. Eventually, however, if ignored, chronic conditions may start to appear. They can ultimately compromise your health, increase the risk of disease, and eventually take you under.

If history teaches us anything, the message should be clear; we will never fulfill every single thing we ever desire. So how can we reduce or eliminate the ramifications that may follow the aftermath of a long-awaited, unfulfilled desire?

We've all heard the axiom "inherent in every desire lies the mechanics to fulfill that desire." This means that every desire is pregnant with the wherewithal to fulfill that desire. To set a desire in motion, all you need to do is to get involved and take action.

That, however, is all you can do to bring it to fruition. Nature will then take over as its sole moderator and become the cocreator in the process of manifestation.

In this world, human beings are bound to the law of action; they must act, but for some reason, they can never completely control the outcome of that action. The delivery of the outcome is the work of nature. When you act and put your heart into what you desire to do, nature will take over and deliver the outcome for you.

So, free from the chains that beg to bind you to the outcome of your desire, act to express that desire. Set the wheels of desire in motion; refrain from being impatient, from throwing tantrums or causing a commotion. In due time, you are bound to enjoy the fruits of your intention. Avoid expecting a predefined outcome; that just puts nature under a lot of limitations. Let nature decide how to best manifest the fruit of your intention.

A great way to streamline this process is to align your desires with the flow of nature. Ideally, this means that your desires should be of a selfless nature. They should potentially benefit not only you but everyone and everything that exists in nature.

Do your desires have the means and the potential to support the balance of nature? Or are they all of a selfish nature? All desires are meant to be fulfilled, especially when they support the flow of nature.

Looking at things from this perspective, you are not only aligning yourself with nature but also avoiding the issues that may arise from forcing things against the flow of nature. When you force nothing and give everything without being attached to your limited concepts, you can be sure that you will live a life filled with health, vitality, and happiness.

DWELL IN THE NOW

Let go of the shadows of the past; shed the anxiety that consumes your flesh, thinking about what may come to pass. Strive to live in the present moment. Being in the present moment keeps you thriving with new life.

The past is gone, the future has not yet come; don't you want to enjoy creating new experiences here and now? When you live in the present moment, you gain a much deeper appreciation of your own higher self. The present is the only time you can unmask that unfettered expression of your intimate inner self.

As you begin to cultivate the art of present-moment awareness, you become consciously aware of not only the physical but also the emotional, spiritual, and mental aspects of your higher self. This form of awareness inherently allows you to harness your inner flow of creativity and freely express yourself.

The present is the only authentic moment that your animating source of life can ever be possibly alive. This very moment is the only time that really ever matters; it's the only fleeting time you are truly alive.

Living in the present moment naturally dissolves the chains that bind you to your mundane routines. Mindless routines encourage supine acceptance of a life that at best fulfills someone else's dreams.

Blind routines often keep you from pursuing your own lifelong ambitions and worthy dreams. Learn to stay in the present moment; become aware of your role in creating your surroundings. Force yourself out of your dull routines.

Avoid the traps of mindless living. Beware of the lure of passive thinking. Embrace the moment; interrupt the cycle of monotony, boredom, and discontent. Condition yourself to become inherently aware and inwardly conscious of the present moment.

Live every day as if it's the last day of your life. Try to stay conscious; try to live a purposeful life. When you are mentally absent in the present moment, you might as well close your eyes, because you are practically neglecting all the wonderful chance occurrences that may present themselves in disguise. Mindful awareness clears up your mental fog; it keeps you healthy and removes your mental block.

When you live in the present moment, you can't help but feel fully conscious; you can't help but feel alive. You feel healthy; you just simply glow with the zest of life.

On the other hand, when you slip away from the bloom of the present moment, you are either rehearsing the memories of the past or worrying about the fate tomorrow may cast. Inherent in this mental trap, you have no choice but to find yourself in bondage. You become quarantined in a house that's walled off with glass.

By reliving the memories of the past or fearing what the future may cast, you are paving yourself a self-destructive path. When you keep dwelling in the past, your painful memories will keep resurfacing as if you are haunted by the past.

Regardless, whether your memories are good or bad,

if you keep living in the past, you hinder your chances of living a passionate life. If you keep thinking about what tomorrow may hold, your anxious thoughts will literally place your life on hold.

Painful memories and anxious thoughts have a tendency to trigger toxic emotions that can cause serious harm. These toxic emotions have the power to circulate toxic substances in your body and eventually cause it harm.

Physiologically speaking, with accumulated toxins circulating in your blood, your cells and organs can eventually get damaged or become permanently scarred. When these cells stop working properly, they reproduce accordingly and create abnormal cells that remember those same hurtful scars.

Dwelling in the memories of the past or living fearfully, in anticipation of the dreaded things that may come to pass, can eventually cause diseases and disorders that impair people's lives. They can cause a variety of unsuspecting conditions like random physical complaints, flulike symptoms, or even more serious conditions that may result in debilitating or disabling scars.

Why would you knowingly do this to yourself? Wake up from your waking dream. Feel the flow of life; feel the rapture of the moment, the only moment you can ever be alive. Nourish your body in the goodness of the moment. Become aware of yourself and your surroundings. Live your precious moments in the everlasting *now*.

Some believe that awareness is a continuum that encompasses not only the daytime and waking states but also the nighttime sleeping and dreaming states. They believe that an enlightened person is indeed awake in the background in all states.

As a matter of fact, a subset of those who subscribe to the ideology of reincarnation believe that the practice of present-moment awareness is the most appropriate preparatory exercise for postmortem awareness. According to this teaching, depending on its state of awareness, a passing soul that's been separated from the body can either be consciously liberated or lost in the "bardo" of death. The word "bardo" refers to an intermediary state, where a soul can either move on or once again get caught up in the cycles of birth and death.

Do you remember how, as a child, you thought that each day seemed to last at least a year? Do you remember how you had so much time in the day to do anything you would want? What happened to all that time?

Does it seem like you are just zooming through your days without being able to get anything done? If you think time is moving faster, you are not alone. As a matter of fact, as strange as it may seem, this time anomaly becomes reliably more noticeable as we transition out of childhood and forget to naturally appreciate the stillness the moment may hold.

You see, the relative fact that you think time is moving faster is not an external occurrence at all. This realization is an internal observation. It becomes more noticeable when you subconsciously choose to ignore the present moment.

It becomes more prominent when you carelessly choose to spend more time dwelling in the past or future. Children, it appears, have a higher tendency to live in the present moment. As a result, they seem to have all the time they could ever want.

For most people, directing the attention to the present moment is not a difficult thing at all. Invariably, it's trying to stay there, where most people stumble and fall.

How can you constantly stay in this present moment when there are so many things that need your attention, so many things that keep you in thrall? Given the way the adult mind is conditioned, staying consciously aware of the present moment is a tricky task that's often easier said than done.

We often have a strong tendency to easily get distracted. Regardless of what we do or where we are, there is always something that threatens to grab our attention and consume our thoughts. In fact, at times we may find it extremely difficult to focus our thoughts.

We can always keep reminding ourselves to stay alert of course, but experience shows that, for many, this strategy is often futile and utterly ineffective. It seems such blatant, head-on attempts almost invariably get drowned and placed in the background by our ordinary day-to-day life events.

Given the complex circuitry of a mature human mind, staying aware of the present moment, moment by moment, is like trying to put a limit on the boundaries of an expanding universal mind. This is no doubt a task that is far beyond the reach of the average human mind.

Therefore, present-moment awareness does not necessarily imply a moment-by-moment accounting of things. Rather, it's an overall attempt to stay aware of the texture and the fabric of one's internal experiences and subjective states. When refined, this strategy can help us grow happier, stay healthier, and achieve our best.

Living in the moment allows you to transform your health and rejuvenate yourself. It allows you to recharge your mind and body with the breath of life. It's only in the present moment when you can heal your body and refresh your mind. The magic inherent in the present moment has the power to cure or at least prevent the diseases that constantly threaten to ravage your body and entangle your mind.

How can you stay constantly focused in the present moment? There are plenty of strategies to draw from of course. For starters, you can consciously learn to channel your streams of thought by choosing activities that provoke personal curiosity and awe. Naturally, when something appeals to your interests, there is a higher likelihood that you would subconsciously remain in the present moment to enjoy it all.

Moreover, try doing things you have never done before. Look for opportunities to express yourself like you never have before. Have you ever traveled to a land where you thought the people, places, and cultures were different from those you are accustomed to? What did it feel like? Were you aware? Did you feel alive? That's the lens through which you should view your daily life if you want to feel alive.

You must revisit the people, places, and customs that surround you in a different light. You must constantly explore new opportunities and find new ways to experience your seemingly ordinary, day-to-day life. This is how you can be aware and consciously grow in life.

Learn to meditate; learn to go within and explore ever new dimensions of your higher self. The space you step into when you truly learn to meditate is none other than the heart of awareness itself. It's a natural place where your mind can remain in touch with your higher self. In time, this meditative sense of awareness begins to permeate your day. It will keep you in the present moment the natural way.

Sometimes, for some people, it may feel too abstract to just think of the present moment. If that's the case for you, then try to maintain awareness by being mindful of something you can outwardly relate to. For example, if you can place a sentimental or memorable object in your purse or pocket, by periodically pulling it out and holding it in your hand, you are automatically reminding yourself to seize the moment and be aware.

Every time you reach for this object, you are literally raising a sign that says you are aware. In this exercise, it would be preferable if the object has some sort of an emotional significance. It would be more powerful, for example, if it somehow reminded you of an important person, an important thing, or an important day.

If that idea does not resonate with you, try imagining a globe of light in the region of the heart, the navel, or immediately above the crown of your head. Keep that awareness as you go about doing the things you do throughout the day. if you can constantly keep that awareness, you are automatically in the present moment; you are dwelling in the present-moment consciousness.

Another effective technique involves the use of memory. This approach ideally focuses on using the power of *prospective* memory to induce awareness. Prospective memory? Yes, developing a prospective memory is a means of training the mind to remember to notice things.

The idea is to preemptively take notice of the repetitive events or common objects we periodically encounter throughout the day. This way we can use them as anchors to trigger our awareness in a systematic way. Ideally, this method should increase our chances of "remembering to be aware" throughout the day.

In this model, we need to create a short list of things we invariably do or encounter each and every day. Whether we want to or not, we seem to consistently do certain things without question every day.

Actions like turning the light switch on or off, checking the clock, going to the bathroom, eating, drinking, or looking at ourselves in the mirror are things that we all inattentively do every day. In addition, we regularly encounter certain situations or contexts, like hearing the dogs bark, listening to the birds chirp, or noticing bicycles, pets, airplanes, or certain colors or models of cars, throughout the day.

We can take advantage of these recurring events and

elements by creating and memorizing a reasonably small list of them and then conditioning ourselves to become aware of them throughout the day. For example, you can remember to give yourself a nudge every time you flick a light switch, every time you hear a dog bark, or every time you see a door that is painted red. Personalize this exercise your way. If done correctly, this can significantly boost your awareness and help you live more attentively every day.

In fact, by using this method, you can sooner or later teach yourself to become aware of the toxic emotional triggers that normally tend to ambush you throughout the day. By becoming aware of these triggers, you can take steps to diffuse them in the present moment, before they can threaten to overwhelm your body or cause disease in any way.

Another powerful method is to mentally verbalize where you are and what you are doing periodically throughout the day. For example, if you are in the kitchen, then silently become aware and acknowledge that you are in the kitchen.

When you move to another location, mentally verbalize where you are right then. Identify the location and the nature of your activity all the time. The only catch is that every time you verbalize it, you need to stop and *feel* the present moment. You need to acknowledge that you are awake and aware there and then.

Track your location and activity all day long. Like a Global Positioning System, internally track and acknowledge your location and activities as you go along. As strange as this may sound, it will finally make sense when you discover that in time, you become much more aware of yourself in space and time. Your mind becomes less distracted; it becomes less confined and restricted.

Another way is to give yourself a purpose, a meaning, a goal, or a mission to accomplish in life. Having a mission in life keeps you awake; it keeps you vibrantly alive. It helps you constantly breathe with new life. A solid purpose keeps you consciously in tune with the stream of life.

Finally, adopt an attitude of gratitude. Look for things and opportunities to be thankful for. This is quite helpful, because when you do, you literally animate the world around you and make it interact with you. This interaction undoubtedly awakens you.

In truth, the possibilities are endless; the ways in which you can stay aware are practically numberless. It must be emphasized, however, that in this process the most important factor in achieving success is the level of motivation and effort one displays in making progress.

BE HAPPY

Close your eyes; observe a moment of silence. What do you feel? Are there any sensations you may be faintly aware of inside? Is there any chance you may feel at least a drop of joy inside?

Is there anything you can do or even think of that would help you feel a tinge of happiness inside? Happiness is a natural state of being; if you don't feel it, is it possible that you may be doing something to mask it or make it hide? Inner joy tends to create a highly magnetic field around you; it attracts others with similar sentiments and draws all the favorable forces of nature on your side.

In joy, you see the world in a different light. Dull colors come to life, relationships blossom, and people become channels through which you can declare and share your experience of joy in life. Joy transforms your dreaded chores into literal works of beauty, acts of charity, and gifts of love. It turns a mere drab existence into a life of beauty, a celebration of splendor, a happy song of harmony and love.

The essence of joy shows its unmarred presence when a child bursts into laughter for no reason at all. Her aura of happiness radiates out in all directions, fills the air, and touches everyone's heart.

Happiness glows like the sun's rays; it reaches out and touches the farthest corners of the universe. It is a beacon of undeniable expression that indescribably quenches everyone's thirst. Like a fountain that wells up from a spring on the mountaintop, the nectar of joy can only roll back over itself and nourish everything on its path with the sweet flow of life.

Happiness is a godsend, a serendipitous blessing, a bounty you can firmly rely on to nourish you for the rest of your days. It is the open secret of the fountain of youth, the binding spell that can magically teleport you to the land of health, wealth, and youth.

The internal echoes of happiness yield amazing effects. To be sure, these effects are not just limited to a mere feeling of bliss. Biologically, they have the potential to revitalize the body and rejuvenate the cells.

In those who find and open the doorway to happiness, the neurohormonal changes that take place can bring about a host of beneficial effects. These changes have the potential to promote health and nourish the body in untold ways. In order for these changes to take place, however, one needs to maintain a firm foundation of inner happiness.

Unfortunately, for most people, a steady state of happiness is not necessarily commonplace. In general, to many, happiness can only be solicited by a cause or a secondary stimulus. In other words, if there is no reason, it makes no sense to even feel a single ounce of happiness.

What most people fail to see is that the kind of happiness that is triggered by an external source has no sustaining, long-term effects. Its impact is often short-lived and temporary. The feelings it unwinds are transitory; the effects are often fleeting and momentary. This kind of happiness can often quickly turn into grief, anguish, despair, and anxiety.

In this world, we live in a whirlwind of circumstances that often changes directions midair. Those who choose to ride out this whirlwind often find themselves thrashing about hither and tither, gasping for air. If we let our moods swing with the fluctuating circumstances, we are constantly doomed to experience alternate feelings of happiness and despair.

When happiness depends on something that is outside of you, it has no sustaining energy to heal you. This form of happiness is transient; it cannot nourish or fortify you. Therefore, the biological changes it stands to create have very little chance of healing you.

True happiness is not caused by anything "out there." It all originates "in here," in your heart, do you hear? It is independent of the turbulent conditions out there.

What is your take on happiness? Are you generally a happy person? If not, is there anything that's keeping you from experiencing inner happiness? Do you need to reevaluate your life choices? Perhaps, it may be wise to give yourself time to rediscover some of the hidden truths you've been ignoring about yourself. Perhaps you need to remember the imprint that is embedded in the DNA of your joyful inner self.

Happiness naturally unfolds its petals when you get back in touch with the essence of your inner self. What's keeping you from living a joyful life? Is there anything you may be withholding from yourself? How do you normally treat yourself? Do you usually take good care of yourself? Do you love yourself? If not, it's time you discovered the pure love that lies dormant in the hidden chambers of your higher self.

Try to get back in touch with the love you keep hidden within your heart. Unconditional love is guaranteed to bring pure joy to your heart. Love is like a sieve that filters out all the impurities of the heart. It disperses the clouds and lets you feel the joy you so yearn for in your heart. Unconditional love cultivates happiness by unweaving the entanglements of the heart.

Try to love others; silently love even those who seemingly cause you unsolicited strain or unnecessary harm. Loving others (regardless of who they are) by decree brings joy to your heart. If this is a new concept to you, don't worry; the exact instructions lie dormant in your heart.

A genuine feeling of gratitude is another treasure that can bring a tremendous amount of joy to your heart. Try to feel thankful for everything you see around you. The miracle of thanksgiving has the power to transform you. It can rekindle that dim spark of happiness inside you. The blissful feelings it stands to unleash promise to help revitalize and rejuvenate you.

Silently praise others; praise even those who may seemingly dislike you. If you feel uncomfortable at first, think nothing of it; just do it anyway. The healthful benefits of it are just a few tiny steps away.

Respect people; be courteous of other's needs. Be kind with your words, requests, and deeds. Regardless of how others have treated you, help them as if you are catering to your own needs. Your kindness will be reciprocated, regardless of their immediate deeds. This will heal you just as effectively as expressing devotion with prayer beads.

This world is like a spider's web: the slightest vibration in any remote part of its matrix affects the whole grid. If your vibrations are composed of love, gratitude, and respect, the whole grid vibrates to the tune of that same effect. So by praising others, by loving people, by giving thanks, and by being kind, you are in effect praising yourself, you are loving yourself, you are thanking and being kind to yourself. Can you see the amazing effect this may have on your states of happiness and health?

You must realize that good or bad, your thoughts, words, and deeds have no choice but to boomerang back and generously slap you right in the back. When reflected back from the mirror of the universe, kind, loving, and thankful thoughts, words, and deeds are rewarded with an inner joy that bursts with healing beams.

So in the end, to get back in touch with your joyful inner self, you need to ultimately create joy for the entire universe, not just yourself. You need to praise others and share your love with them. You need to give thanks for all the experiences you share with them. After all, your inner self is the same universal self that is also shared by them. Therefore, to feel joy from the inside out, you need to first fortify them.

Praising and loving others when they are set against you may seem like a hard thing to do at first. Here, common sense may seem to be missing at first, but it becomes mindlessly clear when you realize that everyone and everything in this world is but a drop in an ocean that is inseparable from yourself.

We all depend on one another, you know; you can never really be completely independent. The boundary that separates you from others is nothing but a mirage that, on close examination, miraculously vanishes and disappears.

In reality, each and every one of us is but a cell that works in conjunction with others to make up the fabric of this universe. The slightest tension anywhere in this fabric causes strain in the overall picture; it affects all its constituents.

The mirage of individuality is just that: a mirage. Everything you do in this world has a consequence that is felt in the farthest corners of the universe. This paradox eventually becomes clear when you finally realize that this universe in its entirety is ultimately a part of your own intimate self.

The people you see around you reflect nothing but the images in the mirror you see yourself through. Everything you think, say, or do travels the length of the distance between you and the people's reflection of you.

You see, you are the totality of the universe; the world begins and ends in you. Once you realize this, you will know that everyone you see around you is nothing but a reflection of you. Inherent in this truth, you can't help but find that eternal everlasting joy that's been kept bottled up inside you.

BE GRATEFUL

Gratitude, some say, is the gateway to heaven. It is one of the basic pillars of strength in every religion. In gratitude, one is mindfully acknowledging the joy of receiving. This inner joy somehow silently evokes the magical process of healing.

Biologically speaking, a genuine sense of gratitude can potentially release endogenous endorphins or "happy substances" in the bloodstream. When these substances uninterruptedly circulate and bathe our tissues, they have the potential to energize and revitalize every cell, every organ, and every sinew.

The healing effect that naturally takes place as a result of adopting a sincere and consistent attitude of gratitude is often far more lasting than that of any manufactured drug in any order of magnitude. Gratitude is like a potion that helps nourish every living cell. It promotes peace, harmony, health, healing, and well-being in the core of every cell.

If you can consistently radiate your grateful feelings out into the far edges of the universe, you will wake up some fine morning to find that the universe has kick-started the whole process in reverse. This newfound bliss can only add to your satisfaction and happiness. Happiness in turn sets the right foundation for a life that overflows with the promise and the gift of vitality and health.

The vibrations of gratitude attract like-minded people to your life. They attract magical encounters, wholesome habits, loving friends, and life situations that are conducive to sustained, long-term health. Therefore gratitude is a key contributing factor in healing or improving one's health.

The attitude of gratitude is one of the most important ingredients in building a strong foundation for health. Once you realize this, you'll no longer hesitate to make it a routine part of your daily life.

How does gratitude help in the process of healing? The mantra is in the practice of appreciating. Regardless of what it is you are appreciating, it's the vibration of gratitude that does the actual work of healing. The attitude of gratitude somehow carries a certain set of vibrations that infallibly aid in the process of healing.

If you are not healthy right now, why not set off the vibes by wholeheartedly delving into the practice of appreciating? You don't have much to be grateful for? Think for a moment; can you acknowledge the air you breathe? Can you appreciate the water you drink? Can you be thankful for the bread you eat? There is an endless number of things you can be thankful for indeed.

Is there anyone you may love, care about, or for whom you may have the slightest feeling? Can you be grateful for your family? Can you be grateful for your freedom, for your life, or your safety? Have you forgotten to appreciate these things?

Do you by any means consider yourself a grateful being? Or do you find it difficult to naturally appreciate things? One way or another, regardless of who you are or what you've been through, it should be practically impossible to ignore how the universe always manages to help you.

Does it feel like the process of healing is a challenging thing? Start being grateful for your health, even though at the moment you might be ill or even potentially suffering. In fact, this is where the magic comes in.

You see, gratitude is nothing but a feeling; it's an impression, a perception, an emotion that is essentially untouched by the passage of time. With gratitude, time is of no essence. This means that the effect it may produce can remain unchanged, regardless of whether your feelings of gratitude pertain to a person, an event, or a thing in the present, the future, or the past.

In fact, the most amazing property of the exercise of gratitude is its timeless nature. You see, its healing potential lies coiled up in this timeless feature. It can produce a fast-forward effect and speedily heal you by the virtue of its timeless nature. When it comes to healing, this can be the single most valuable piece of information you can ever possibly find in your favor.

Here, the secret behind the promise of healing lies in the art of prematurely appreciating. In essence, the feeling of being thankful for things in advance creates a shift in the way we would expect to see things unfold in our lives. Giving thanks in advance helps you align your desires with the realities you wish to see in your mind. In this process, if health is what you so desire, then that's exactly what you'll find.

One way or another, we are all doing this without really

consciously realizing how or which way. Why not take advantage of this age-old wisdom and let it play out our way?

Believe it or not, this mind trick in essence mobilizes your subconscious mind to set the stage and arrange your affairs in a way that will create the realities you wish to experience someday. This is not superstition; it's not science fiction; it is a well-documented fact.

The only catch is that you would actually have to involve your emotions. You would have to generate an explosive internal feeling that's strong enough to genuinely support your expression of gratitude for health and healing.

Therefore, it would not be nearly as effective if you just simply verbalized your sense of thankfulness for this or that. You would actually have to use your scale of emotions to *repeatedly and consistently* demonstrate what your state of health should be like in your mind. As you continue to express your feelings of gratitude, you would have to consistently see yourself bubbling with health and glowing with the zest of life.

The ultimate catalyst here is a *persistent* inward expression of a bursting emotion. Therefore, if you want to set things in motion, you need an unconditional commitment to engage your emotions.

The idea is simple: *feeling* grateful for an event before it has physically taken place can trick your brain into thinking that you have already observed that experience somewhere in your memory, some way. Sooner or later, your subconscious mind will create the appropriate circumstances for you to experience it anyway.

FORGIVE YOURSELF

Believe it or not, all too often, many of the chronic or debilitating conditions people face may be traced back to an old, unresolved, adverse, or traumatic experience in life. A long-held grudge, an act of hatred, a perpetual source of anger, an old unforgiven act or injury, or a culture of fear can all either cause or at least contribute to one's ill health.

It's not all that uncommon for an unresolved history of crisis, dilemma, dispute, or conflict to initiate a legacy of unhealed psychological scars. If left unresolved, these unhealed scars can subconsciously turn into depression, addiction, anxiety, malnutrition, poor health, or other diseases or physical flaws.

Growing up, we all tend to accumulate and hold on to such undesirable scars. We somehow seem to have a peculiar tendency to hold on to such problematic, negatively charged emotions and thoughts. Somehow, instead of finding a way to resolve them, we assimilate and store them in our bodies by leaving them suspended in the womb of time.

These unresolved scars have a remarkable ability to snowball, change, and mutate into practically every sort of disease and disorder known to humankind. In truth, these diseases and disorders may be nothing but the crystallized manifestation of our unsettled, unresolved feelings and disharmonious thoughts.

In reality, though consciously inconceivable, this

is the means by which many of our diseases and disorders inwardly take root and work from the inside out. Regretful memories and past mistakes have a tendency to turn up from time to time and create internal tides. Time and again, the sheer pain that gets triggered by these memories leaves a cloud of dust that obscures the original source of discomfort and disgust.

Though in time we may consciously forget the original source of these emotional scars, we end up carrying the residual memory of their wounds in our subconscious minds. In time, the sticky residues that linger from having experienced these emotional scars tend to manifest in the form of a morbid or a chronic condition that ultimately taints the wholesome experience of life.

Although by this point, seeking medical care may pay the highest dividends by far, to alleviate our chronic conditions once and for all, we need to pacify the primary disturbances that usually start them all. What are these disturbances? What else but the lingering memories of those unhealed scars.

The most effective way to resolve these scars is to "forgive and forget." Notice that the first step is to *forgive*. Without forgiving, you will never be able to forget. In this process, you need to forgive all the parties that may be possibly involved in forming that scar. Incidentally, this includes *you*.

You see, the reason you are suffering from many of the discomforts, diseases, and disorders that keep you in thrall is because you are unable to forgive yourself for all the painful memories that remain unresolved. To once and for all rid yourself of the maladies that hunt you in your life, you need to learn to forgive everyone, including *yourself*.

Forgetting the past when you can't forgive yourself has no value in healing at all. You need to first forgive yourself before you can truly begin to heal not only psychologically but also physically.

Self-forgiveness is the greatest healing balm of them all. The caveat, however, is that self-healing is not possible until you also forgive all the parties involved. You see, you will never be able to forgive yourself until you have learned to forgive all. That's right; the cost of the cure is the ability to forgive all. This for most people is the hardest thing to come to terms with overall.

I once read the act of forgiving is like spreading the seeds of love. In love, all the differences, pains, and disharmonies ultimately dissolve. Forgiveness therefore is the key to healing; it is one of the greatest healing secrets of them all.

But how can you forgive those who have hurt you and have no remorse for what they have done? This is where most people get blindsided, thinking that their painful memories are caused by others, when, in reality, they themselves were the ones that created them all.

You see, you are the creator of all your experiences. Like the people and the figures in a nighttime dream, you animate the people, the situations, and the circumstances in your daytime, waking dream.

Painful or not, *you* are the only one responsible for creating your life experiences. Others merely follow the scripts you keep writing all along. If you can't see the connection, it's because you are somehow unable to connect the dots and follow along.

Invariably, by blaming others for your experiences, you are expressly blaming yourself. Therefore, the best way to find relief from your ailing circumstances is to forgive all the parties involved. Only then will you ever be able to truly forgive yourself and neutralize your unhealed scars. You may never forget the memory of your old scar, but once you forgive yourself and all the parties involved, your memory will no longer hurt you or cause physical harm.

The fact of the matter is that an emotional scar is a life lesson that you have not yet learned to master at all. That's why it has turned into a physical ailment or scar. It will begin to heal on its own when you learn to let go of your destructive feelings and forgive all. This process of forgiveness must entail an inward surrender and letting go of your anger, blame, shame, fear, regret, bitterness, resentment, or any negative sentiment that may involve you and any other person near or far.

When done genuinely, the act of forgiveness has the power to melt away your emotional knots. In time, it can restore your well-being, and allow you to experience a tremendous peace of mind.

Remember, just the same way your chronic physical ailments took time to take root, so will healing need time to give your long-standing conditions the boot. This is where true forgiveness requires enough patience to show the beauty of its fruit.

LOVE YOURSELF

Regardless of who you are, what you do, or where you are from, you need a healthy body to discover your true potential in life. Without a healthy body, you won't have enough zeal to thoroughly experience the zest of life.

It makes perfect sense to reason that a healthy body should start with a sensible diet, moderate physical activity, and a balanced emotional and psychological life. Though essential, however, none of these, either individually or combined, can be comprehensive enough to support a healthy foundation in life. The secret glue that fills the cracks and strengthens the foundation is the art of cultivating the light of self-love.

Without loving yourself, you will never achieve that healthy inner glow of life. Loving yourself does not have to imply an egotistic, self-absorbed, or narcissistic way of life. Instead, it can be a means of recognizing and respecting the true essence and value of your higher self.

This higher self, when finally perceived, will add a new perspective to the meaning of life. This inner self is the same point of reference that is literally shared with every animate and inanimate object in life. In loving and respecting this inner self, you are indeed loving and respecting all of life. In this state, you are in tune with that harmony that is sacredly shared by all of life. Only then, only when in tune, can you ever hope to enjoy the nectar of a healthy life.

Unfortunately, most people are either unaware of, or at least misunderstand, the value of this inner self.

Conditioned by the battles and the wounds they have experienced in life, they seem to constantly disapprove of or harshly criticize themselves. In fact, many find it difficult to look in the mirror without experiencing the agony of judgment, revulsion, guilt, shame, or disgust.

The tragedy is that these feelings and emotions are physically harmful. They create a toxic cloud that undermines the health of the body. By nature, they have a great tendency to agitate the immune system and weaken the body.

To better understand this concept, it may be helpful to remember that our bodies are composed of cells that cluster together to form tissues, organs, and systems. What's important to understand is that these cells, organs, and systems are not functionally integrated by themselves. They exist to serve the body, and, as such, to one degree or another, they are ruled by the dictates of the conscious and the subconscious minds.

Just the same way the citizens and the authorities of cities, counties, and states in a country secure the benefits of a united government, so the cells, the organs, and the systems of the body, to one degree or another, follow the dictates or the anchored inclinations of an intelligent, creative mind.

By default, then, to follow the lead of a unifying mind, these cells, organs, and systems have the cognitive apparatus to dynamically eavesdrop on the internal thoughts, moods, and feelings that occupy one's mind. Somehow, they have the ability to monitor or listen in on the thoughts, images, and conversations that take place in one's mind.

Though there are plenty of subconscious safeguards, if these internal thoughts, moods, feelings, and conversations are consistent or intense enough, they can make a lasting impression on the organic mirror of the mind. Our cells then have the capability to respond to these impressions by activating pathways that create physically toxic or healing environments. In time, these internal conditions and environments can naturally lead to health, healing, happiness, or disease, decrepitude, and wretchedness.

Naturally, with undesirable impressions, our bodies may suffer ailments and maladies, ranging from minor afflictions to major physical or emotional disturbances. Therefore, the way we intimately see and treat ourselves can greatly affect the way we look, the way we feel, or the way we would respond to the threat of these internal environments.

Our family members, schoolteachers, peers, and others often play an important role in shaping the groundwork that underlies our toxic monologues and faulty self-images. Often, years of negative conditioning make it difficult to break the cycles that perpetuate these negative thoughts and faulty images.

This is exactly why it's so important to love yourself. When you learn to love yourself, you will dissolve the negative emotions with which you bind yourself; you will begin to heal and revitalize yourself. Inner love helps you cultivate a genuine sense of self-worth. It generates a feeling of harmony and happiness, which naturally paves the road for a successful start.

Therefore, before you can truly experience the natural wonder of health and vitality, you need to learn to love yourself; you need to stop being critical of yourself. Self-love is an essential nutrient in the recipe that promotes harmony, health, and happiness.

No one can describe what love is. Like the invisible, subatomic particles that leave no trace, love mysteriously manages to evade our external senses. In love, there is a sweet, intoxicating sense of immortal bliss. When the tidal wave of self-love hits, it makes you wonder why you've never tasted anything like this. Yet, when it hits, there is absolutely no ambiguity about what self-love is.

The jolt of self-love is an awakening that resembles a divine kiss. It cleanses your body, purifies your heart, and washes your sins. How can you love yourself like this? By stepping into that silent space of inner awareness.

Finding self-love is a journey of self-discovery. This journey is best traveled when you are all alone. It calls for frequent intervals of introspection and self-reflection, all on your own.

Unfortunately, many people find it downright frightening to be quiet and all alone. They must always live and do things in the company of others, or they will never get anything done on their own. The urge to rely on others is sometimes so strong, some may find it difficult to even breathe alone.

When incidentally on their own, some may feel a strong urge to keep themselves occupied with distractions. If they don't, they will go crazy being on their own.

They feel a compulsory need to watch TV, listen to music, or talk on the phone.

To love yourself, you must first get to know yourself. You must face your fears and make peace with yourself. Think for a moment; can you honestly say that you are an unshakable source of love for yourself? Stand in front of a mirror and examine the reflection of your self. Short, tall, obese, skinny, graceful, or not, can you honestly say that you truly love yourself?

In most cases, it's not what you see in the mirror that gets in your way; it's your own misconceptions that keep your precious love so far away. Start by telling yourself that you love yourself. Stand in front of a full-sized mirror and praise yourself. Praise your own image as you say all the good things you want to see manifest in yourself.

Confidently affirm all the good qualities you want to see in yourself. Talk to yourself; say all the good things you can possibly say to yourself. Say how good you are, say how wonderful you are, say how much you love yourself. Say it even if in the beginning you don't feel that way about yourself.

Create a list of all the good qualities you would like to see in yourself. When you do, resolve to tirelessly reaffirm them to yourself. See yourself infused with strength, youth, health, and natural energy. Imagine yourself glowing with a timeless sense of vitality. Imagine loving yourself for all eternity.

Again, in case you are wondering, this is not a quick fix; it's not a part-time thing; it's a way of life. It requires a commitment that extends far beyond what anyone can expect in the context of day-to-day life. Just fake it till you make it. Go on blindly assuming that you truly love yourself. If all this seems strange, just ask yourself: with the way things are, are you happy with the way you've managed these things for yourself?

If you stick with it, in time you will begin to develop the confidence, courage, and ability to believe in yourself. Eventually, your relentless efforts to unselfishly love yourself will begin to predominate and translate into a force that will help you rediscover your true love for your inner self.

Love begets love, you know; on awakening, your unpretentious love for yourself will radiate out from the center of your heart and become a magnet that attracts universal love. You will by default attract the kind of love that matches the vibrations that emanate from the innocent chords of your own heart.

Your love for yourself will change you, transform you, and touch everyone else around you. In love, pains dissipate, illnesses dissolve, obstacles vanish, and hardships fall. Your love for yourself will eventually grow to not only nourish you but the whole world around you.

True self-love is not a selfish thing at all. It is the most unselfish gift you can give yourself from the bottom of your heart. True self-love not only affects you but also everyone else around you. It encourages harmony and beautifies the world around you. It's a win-win situation for everyone, not just you.

In love, you can't help but feel fulfilled. When you love

yourself, you openly exude a radiant glow and develop a sense of inner peace. So be good to yourself. Love yourself if you want these things.

HAVE HOPE

In its most elemental essence, hope is nothing but a desirable feeling of expectation. What's amazing is that this mere feeling of expectation is a volatile substance that can ignite the spark of creation. Give yourself the gift of hope. Expect something wonderful. Expect something good.

Hope casts a spell with which you can capture the core substance of your desired goal. Hope simply empowers the soul. It gives your soul the energy to thrust forward and flatten all the bumps and the hurdles that may lie ahead on the surface of the road.

The power of hope is so mysterious, it can cheat death, cure the incurable, or unearth the unbelievable. Hope is the light that leads people out of despair. It's the wind that blows away the mist and clears the air. Decorate your thoughts with the glory of hope.

No matter what the circumstances, no matter what your fate, be a hopeful soul. Believe in yourself; bend the rules in your favor by being hopeful. Expect a magical cure. When your hope is unconditional and pure, the universe will rearrange the stars to create a cure.

BE PURE

Does it seem like having a healthy body is but a distant dream for you? Every little word you mutter and every little thing you do can play an important role in reshaping, reforming, and restructuring the appearance and the outcome of the life you see before you.

When we think of the future and dream a dream, we literally cast a mold for it, in hopes that maybe someday we can realize that dream. What we don't understand, however, is that every casual thought can have a direct effect on shaping and reshaping that dream.

Thoughts carry the essence of the most creative force in life. Like embryonic stem cells, thoughts give form to and create the world we erect around ourselves. Our thoughts are the precise progenitors of the circumstances that help shape our state of health.

For this reason, it is crucial to generate and maintain thoughts that engender a healthy inner life. Unfortunately, however, for the average individual, most such thoughts are often rendered ineffective by uncertainty, fear, and self-doubt.

That's why our lives are often challenged by contradictions, diseases, obstacles, and difficult times. Can you imagine the world if we were but able to completely subdue our unnecessary doubts?

Every time you doubt yourself, you are in effect stepping on the cells of your budding creation; you are literally crushing its foundation. Ironically, people's lives are often plagued by fear, doubt, and hesitation.

We all do this; time after time, we envision glorious castles of victory and pride, but as soon as we lay a few bricks, we recklessly dismantle them with our doubtful, indecisive minds. Time and again, we doubt ourselves, and by doing so, we sever the lifeline that connects our dreams with the creative source.

If you want a strong, healthy, or youthful body, you need to come up with a solid dream that supports that body. Once you do, you need to stick to that vision until you materialize that body. Vacillation, doubt, uncertainty, or indecisiveness are at best deterrents that only serve to weaken your body.

If you choose health, you need to once and for all create that mold and keep it polished with a solid hold. Slay the demons that create doubt with the strength and the power of your purity of thought. By remaining steadfast against all doubts, you can preserve the integrity of your creative thoughts.

If you want a healthy body, create a healthy mold that captivates you. Once you do, never doubt or for any reason look behind you. Trust in the precious purity that innocently exists within you.

CHAPTER 4

The Art of Living

To be healthy, you need to engage yourself. To stay healthy, you need to set rules for yourself; you need to take action and apply yourself. If you want to be healthy, you need to take an active role in caring for yourself; you need to step out of your comfort zone and apply yourself.

Ultimately, your success hinges on your commitment to create a powerful, healthy routine for yourself. More important, if you wish to avoid falling into a yo-yo trap, you need to keep going and continue to motivate yourself.

THE ROLE OF AFFIRMATIONS

Affirmations serve to validate and solidify the realities we wish to perceive in life. They can be verbal, visual, auditory, symbolic, or any way we may normally experience the fullness of life.

They can inadvertently take shape through our imaginations, thoughts, or internal monologues. They can either be self-initiated or imposed on us by our families, friends, colleagues, the media, or community-enforced laws.

When constantly replayed on the back screen of our minds, affirmations tend to keep creating the realities we face in our lives. In truth, affirmations give form to and crystallize the very realities we expect to experience in our lives.

Consciously or not, when we replay the events we have witnessed or perhaps even expect to someday encounter in our minds, we keep reaffirming what we should expect to have happen in our lives. Our seemingly unimportant internal monologues are affirmations that ultimately help determine what we do and who we become in our lives.

In reality, we are all affirmation pros; we mastered this ability in early childhood, before we could even count our toes. Unfortunately, we do it heedlessly, without even knowing the rules or the underlying terms.

Let me ask you this: What goes through your mind when you see your own reflection in the mirror on the wall? Do you like who you are? If you think you are not worthy, then there you are! Remember, pleasant or not, your affirmative thoughts create your realities and define who you are. Your daily unassuming affirmations can mindlessly dictate the quality of the health you experience in your life.

Oftentimes, people can be very critical of themselves. This self-criticism, though seemingly harmless, keeps reaffirming the molds with which they should re-create themselves. Self-criticism can be constructive, but when carried out unremittingly, it can lead to circumstances that may ultimately change destinies and destroy dreams.

Become aware of the habits that unintentionally reinforce your undesirable molds. Once you become aware of these patterns, it should be easy to replace them with affirmations that help you consciously create what your future should hold.

When we become aware of the colossal power our affirmations hold, we become true creators; we become conscious of our own ability to cast our own molds. What sort of qualities would *you* like to shape with your mold? Beauty? Strength? Health? Happiness? Love? Then use affirmations to turn these qualities into lasting molds that can replicate the essences they hold.

Affirmations can help you recondition your mind and ultimately re-create yourself. Most people are familiar with the concept of daily affirmations. Some successfully use it, while others seem to perpetually struggle with it. The most common complaint is that they can't yield consistent results with it.

Some are quick to get excited about it, only to lose

heart and just as quickly drop it. They just can't find any measurable signs of progress with it. In truth, positive or not, affirmations do work. You just need to give the concept a fair chance; you need to stick with it and give it enough time to work.

Affirmations can help purify and reprogram the backbone of your thoughts. They can help you restructure the dynamic model and the trajectory of your life. The only disclaimer is that they won't be as effective if they are taken up as a mere casual exercise.

In reality, positive affirmative thoughts can take you a long way toward breaking your negative habits and changing your destructive thoughts. Truth be told, however, they are not nearly as powerful if they are just lightly entertained or blindly exercised.

Your degree of success when affirming your positive thoughts greatly depends on the magnitude and the intensity of the effort you can altogether dramatize. If you don't challenge yourself, your assertions will never materialize.

To begin with, it is important that your affirmations support a *strong purpose*, an important cause. Naturally of course, your cause should be compelling enough for you to keep affirming and reaffirming what you want.

Is there any one thing in your body you desperately need to improve? To see that desire come through, you need to have an undying conviction, a dedication, a commitment to affirm and reaffirm your desire and your purpose through and through. You need to mentally assert and reassert your desire and purpose as often as it takes for you to finally see it through.

Ideally, your affirmations should be enticing enough to help you replace your negative thoughts. But that's not all; to make them effective, you also need to find a way to break through the mental barriers that safeguard these negative thoughts. Your affirmations need a way to chip away at the barriers that protect your negative thoughts. If they don't get through, they can at best yield temporary results.

Think of the power of affirmations as a sweeping wave of a raging flood. With one surge, they can easily engulf your islands of negative thought. The downside, however, is that a torrent of flood is often short-lived. After the waters recede, you are once again left with your islands of undesirable thought.

If you want results, you need to practice; you need to literally saturate your subconscious mind with affirmative thoughts. If you don't, they will never gain enough traction to help you achieve what you want.

It's the power of practice that helps you chip away at the mental barriers that protect your negative thoughts. Practice refines the form and adds fuel to your affirmative thoughts. It's the crucial step with which you can etch your desired affirmations on the tablet of your subconscious mind.

In addition, to fulfill their function, your affirmations need to be heavily fortified with the language of emotion. They need to be backed by strong feelings. It's the feeling that sets things in motion and helps you yield results.

Your affirmative thoughts therefore should ideally serve you in two ways: they should not only promote pure, wholesome, and healthy thoughts but also effectively drown the islands that support your *negative* thoughts. To truly support this cause, you need a strong purpose, a strong range of emotions, and a practice regimen that can help you reach and replace your unhealthy subconscious thoughts.

THE ROLE OF INTENTION

Intention some say is the most important ingredient in the recipe of creation. Literally, every form of manifestation in this world is by default a product of intention.

In fact, intention is an underlying cause of the wonders of creation. The power of intention defines the unfathomable limits of human potentiality and qualification. It is that magical spark that helps set things in motion.

Intention is the ethereal windmill with which we develop power and motion. It is the quantum wave function with which we individualize the mechanics of creation. When up against the power of intention, this whole universe surrenders, with or without ammunition.

The force of intention is the first impulse that radiates out from the flame of desire. When you have a strong desire, your intention to act on it reflects the force of that desire. The stronger the intention, the higher the likelihood that you will act to realize that desire.

People often underestimate the power of intention. Nevertheless, it's the intention that cranks the wheels of creation. Believe it or not, our span of attention often precludes us from having enough focus to follow the tedious course of creation. Whether we are aware of it or not, however, the process of creation never fails to flow from the smallest thread of intention, all the way through to its manifestation.

In reality, intention is the driving force that builds on the law of manifestation. Without an intention, there is no fuel to crank-start the wheels of creation. It is pure intention that initiates the means of taking action. Without an intention, there is no momentum to take any action.

How can we consciously draw on the power of intention? By enhancing our focus and maintaining concentration. Failure often stems from having too many desires that compete for our undivided attention. This inevitably weakens the power of intention. Without enough focus, we have nothing to work with but an unclear intention. This will make it difficult to reach the desired destination. The driving force behind it is not strong enough to bring the desire into fruition.

What's more, we need the power of a clear and strong purpose to support the force of intention. In many instances, this purpose may need to be adorned with the robe of inspiration. It may need to be counterbalanced by a tone of hope or desperation. In a way, the strength and the degree of inspiration, hope, or desperation can be said to determine the fate of that intention.

Despite all these measures, however, even with a strong purpose and the power of concentration, it may still be difficult to reap the fruit of an intention. To reinforce the creative power of an intention, it may be best to paint it with the vivid colors of emotion.

The power of intention is best harnessed when it's infrastructure is backed by a strong emotion. You see, the potential power of intention is not necessarily realized through conscious thoughts or words alone; it's the feeling that gives the power of intention its meat and bone.

When backed by a strong emotion, an intention readily finds the spark needed to navigate the road to creation. How can you energize your intention with a strong emotion? So far, we've covered a lot of ground in describing the power of emotion in conscious creation. What we've covered up to now of course is tremendously powerful, but let's take it a step further and explore a new horizon.

Remember, emotions jump the gap that bridges the mind-body connection. As such, they are thoughts that are selectively interwoven into the fabric of various organs or body parts. This means that many of our emotions are already potentially stored in these visceral organs or body parts.

Haven't you ever loved someone from the bottom of your heart? What did it feel like? How strong was that bond? I'm sure from time to time, we've all heard people say how they have a "gut feeling" about this or that, or a "chill running down their spine." At one point or another, we've all heard people say how they feel a lump in the throat, joy in the heart, or a sense of queasiness in the stomach, have we not?

It's not all that uncommon for people to describe an emotion while making reference to a certain organ or body part. Have you ever felt a lump of pent-up emotions in your throat? Have you ever felt a sense of oneness, compassion, or love in the region of your heart? Have you ever experienced a sense of fear, power, or anxiety in the stomach, knees, head, or other body parts?

For millennia, people in different cultures have been taught that there are distinct vortices of energy associated with certain body parts. These energy centers seem to have the ability to link our emotions to their physical counterparts.

Westerners often find it unusual to define a connection between emotions and physical body parts. Mounting data, however, is beginning to suggest that there is indeed a connection between emotions and various body parts.

When people talk about a sensation of joy in the heart, they often mean it, because they generally tend to feel that sensation in the region of the heart. When someone says that her heart aches from some tragic news or from depression, jealousy, or loss, she is describing the physical symptoms of an emotional counterpart. When someone says that he feels a knot of fear in his stomach or his heart, he is literally describing an emotional phenomenon that is attached to that body part.

These are strong feelings that are somehow associated with physical organs, nerve bundles (plexuses), or body parts. Strong emotions have the power to mend or break many worlds in your heart. A heartfelt emotion can play a pivotal role in making a sizable donation or helping a colossal cause.

Emotions can ignite patriotic wars, altruistic missions, and community uprisings against certain actions or laws. A feeling of disgust in the area of the gut can tear nations apart. A sense of helplessness in that same region can make a mother jump in front of traffic to save her child from an oncoming car.

Knowing this, it should make sense to try to take advantage of the power these organ-coupled emotions can potentially provide. We can do this by formulating and releasing our intentions from the organs, nerve bundles, or the body parts where these stored emotions tend to naturally reside.

Why not take advantage of our visceral, organ-coupled feelings to supercharge our intentions and thoughts? In this process, we are literally fertilizing the seed of intention by silently verbalizing our intentions through the physical organs where we normally feel our intense emotions. Which organ would this normally be for you?

For most people, strong feelings are subjectively localized in the central trunk, perhaps in the abdomen or in the region of the heart. For some, it's in the area of navel, hands, or other body parts. Others may feel it in the head or in the space between their eyebrows. Where is it for you?

Remember, to intensify your intentions, try to originate and broadcast them from the physical organs or areas you normally take notice of. To do this, you need to be mindful of that organ or body part while setting your intention for what you want. For example, try to project your intention from the bottom of your heart.

Naturally, to induce healing, regeneration, or in the least a vibrant sense of well-being, it would make sense to practice broadcasting or projecting that intention from your strongest organ or body part. If you have yet to develop the visceral acuity to identify that part, try experimenting with an area in your central trunk. For most people, this may be the area of the navel, the stomach, or the heart. As always, if you are truly genuine and seek results, you need to practice, practice, practice; you can't throw a lighthearted shot.

To recap, intention is the force with which we can jump-start the wheels of creation. To fulfill the content of its mission, a seed of intention needs the right foundation. This foundation is supported by the power of purpose, the effect of concentration, and the anatomy of emotion.

Emotions essentially support the ripening of the seed of intention. Subconsciously, we tend to store strong, potential emotions in different energy vortices that are selectively hyperlinked to certain visceral organs and body parts. When we link our intentions to these body parts, we may find it much easier to achieve what we want.

The Role of Intuition

Deep within the heart of each and every one of us, there is an instinctive, visceral impulse of heartfelt awareness that serves to harmoniously guide us along the path of natural evolution and self-realization. This impulse of awareness has often been described in books, tales, and literature by various means, including the sixth sense, telepathy, clairvoyance, clairaudience, or intuition.

For the sake of simplicity, we'll call this impulse intuition. Intuition is that remarkable natural ability of the mind to somehow miraculously perceive knowledge without the interference of the physical senses, logic, or reason.

Intuition describes one's natural ability to tap into that primordial source of accessible knowledge and information. This source is a seeming guide that is always accessible as we blindly make our journey through life. We all feel its presence; some, of course, feel it more than others, but nevertheless, we all have it encrypted somewhere in the fabric of our collective DNA.

This extrasensory power of perception gives us a means through which we can potentially benefit from that singular knowledge that's shared throughout the universe. It's an amazing gift, yet many of us choose to completely ignore it. Others may by chance partially use it, but if they do, it is more often than not used for trivial things. Instead of using it to advance and grow, they choose to try their luck or gamble with nowhere to go.

To most people, intuition is like an unreasonable

hunch. They think of it as an intangible feeling, an impalpable cloud that is too high to touch. In truth, relying on an unreasoning, illogical hunch is a gamble most people are not willing to take.

This is perhaps rightly so, because when ignored or seldom used, intuition is nothing more than a rusty tool. Who would rely on a rusty skill as a basis of information or as a practical tool?

Like a muscle, intuition needs to be constantly used; if it's not, it invariably atrophies through nonuse. If you want to rely on your intuition, you need to use it; you need to cultivate it. Only then can you ever really rely on it as a powerful tool.

Having repressed or ignored our intuitive faculties for generations, most of us humans are no longer able to tell the difference between a sensation and a fair measure of intrinsic intuition. Therefore, we tend to easily dismiss innate feelings and instinctual clues. If you want your sense of intuition to shine and guide you through, you must demand an extrasensory input in everything you do.

Exercise your power of intuition in whatever you set out to do. Learn to act on the basis of intuition in every situation, regardless of what you may encounter, see, or do. Use it to your advantage; never be afraid of trusting what it may bring you.

Trusting your intuition would mean that you trust that inner wisdom that inherently resides within you. To get to that point, however, you need to learn to rediscover the *inner you*. This requires a keen appreciation of the natural qualities that are inherently instilled within you.

To start with, try to take note of the outcomes of your actions and daily decisions. Once you do, ask yourself if these outcomes would have been any different had your intuition guided you through. Notice how your decisions might have changed had you let your sense of intuition step forward and help you.

With practice, your sense of intuition will eventually flourish and shine through. Little by little, as you allow your intuition to flow through, let it gently inspire and guide you. Once you allow your intuition to shine through, you will see that it will do anything within its power to rightfully guide you.

Guided by the intuitive inner you, this whole world will soon beg to unfold before you. When you align yourself with the intuitive values that guide you, you will begin to enjoy life and excel in whatever it is you naturally do. Life suddenly flows smoother; your relationships and interactions become deeper and richer. Your decisions and actions become more effective and more meaningful.

All of this takes a backseat, however, when you finally realize that intuition is a way of harmonizing you body to the tune of nature. When you are truly in tune with the rhythm and the harmony of nature, your body will begin to find its balance by drawing on the intelligence of nature. Somehow, it will inherently know how to exert itself. It will know how to be, when to sleep, when to wake up, when to eat, or what to eat.

With the help of intuition, your body will gradually begin to heal itself. It will begin to naturally restore and rejuvenate itself. All of this suddenly becomes possible when you learn to unclog your channels and get back in touch with your intuitive inner self. All it takes is practice to reawaken this intuitive inner self.

THE ROLE OF EXERCISE

It should be common sense to think that exercise plays an important role in the restoration, preservation, and promotion of health, yet many people go on living without ever taking an extra step to exercise in the name of health. In the old days before the industrial age, people actually earned a living by hands on hunting, sailing, farming, or, simply put, physically working. This physical work unpretentiously accomplished what many of us with sedentary lifestyles wish to strive for today.

The new age of information and technology, however, has for the most part taken the need for physical activity out of the equation. With today's jobs and comfortable lifestyles, moderate physical activity does not always present itself as a favorable occasion.

Regardless of the times, however, moderate physical activity is still an all-in-one conditioning tool. It helps you control your weight, boost your energy, and improve your mood. It's a proactive means of toning your muscles, supporting your joints, and strengthening your bones.

It can help excrete wasteful toxins and revitalize your cells, tissues, and organs. Exercise can pave the way for a vibrant, disease-free life. It can set the stage for a balanced psychological, emotional, and spiritual life.

Physical exercise does not have to be rigorous; it does not need to be overly lengthy or exceptionally strenuous. It certainly should not be chorelike, dull, or tedious. Your skin, internal organs, muscles, and bones all thrive on some form of physical activity, but this activity does not necessarily need to be performed with unnecessary intensity.

To physically flourish, all the body needs is a healthy measure of flexibility. It needs to be gently stressed and stretched beyond its natural tone and pliability. This can be easily accomplished by doing something fun, something that incidentally includes some form of physical activity and exercise that's not overly done.

Do something safe that makes you feel good. It is highly likely that you will stick with your routine if you do something that is exhilarating, something that makes you feel good.

Exercise should be fun; it should be joyful to your senses or else it's not worth attempting at all. If anything, exercise should boost your confidence and clear your mind.

Find a routine that's entertaining and fun. Whether it's a light weight-bearing exercise, a brisk walk, a quick swim, or a quiet jog, make it long enough, and certainly challenging or interesting enough to make you feel like you are having fun.

What is *your* favorite form of exercise? Some enjoy yoga, many prefer group activities, others enjoy dancing, swimming, hiking, biking, running, and so on. If you don't already exercise, find a healthy routine that's fun.

The Role of Diet

Food is literally the plastic material with which we subconsciously construct, nourish, and repair our tissues and cells. Therefore, what we eat indistinctly affects every part of the body, cell by cell. In fact, it not only affects the body but the *mind* as well.

Everyone knows that food gets digested in the gastrointestinal tract. This, however, is only the beginning of its inward journey to be exact. When broken down, its molecules continue to be used by every cell and every organ as a matter of fact.

The body somehow subconsciously extracts all the essential ingredients in food. The beverages, the snacks, the meals, the vitamins, the minerals, the stimulants, or the supplements we lightheartedly ingest, all break down into their elemental components and either get rejected or directed and utilized as cellular food.

The foods we eat not only help supply the building blocks our cells may need but also the much-needed energy our bodies ultimately need. Food has the power to change one's behavior, mood, and physiology.

Your choice of foods can altogether influence the fabric of your consciousness. It seems mind-boggling to think that the average individual may find it hard to believe that food can actually affect the consciousness, but in fact it does.

Coffee and tea, as well as organic, processed, or seemingly friendly foods can have a marked effect on energy, metabolism, and mood. Certain foods, drugs, or beverages, for example, can slur the speech, alter the mentation, or even cause a sense of enhanced perception. Some can help with fatigue. Others can cause a sense of dullness or lethargy. Many can promote a sense of focus, alertness, or mental clarity.

Some can cause flushing, agitation, restlessness, or even anxiety. Others can help trigger depression or even make you feel a deep sense of tranquility. Many can promote a sense of well-being, euphoria, or energy.

Unfortunately, most people are oblivious to the side effects of what they eat. As you can see, however, the body is tremendously influenced by what you eat. This influence is mediated not only by the type of food but also the quality and the quantity of what you eat. Therefore, it is important to be mindful of the foods you eat.

For example, it should be obvious to see how junk foods simply decompose into junk by-products, contaminants, and their residues. By the same token, it should be easy to see how nutritious foods break down into their essential nutrients and nourishing cellular foods. Invariably, however, this is not what most people pay attention to when they think about food. Instead, they think about food in terms of weight control, diet, or energy boost.

They lap up all the trivial things the media feeds them as a part of an economically driven advertising tool. Thanks to social media, people around the world are becoming increasingly obsessed with the next wave of diet that would perhaps promote weight loss or energy boost.

Believe it or not, with or without the help of the media,

none of these concepts is in any way revolutionary or new. They are just old ideas that keep resurfacing with a new point of view.

Diets have been the subject of popular culture since the dawn of the human race. Yo-yo diets have plagued the mind of humanity even before religions began to ban one thing or the next.

Among many popular themes, today's hot ideas include prepackaged calorie-counted foods, designer vitamins, and bottled goods. To add to this, there is a variety of laboratory prepared lipids, proteins, and carbohydrates that are supposed to complement organically labeled foods.

The truth is that none of these foods has ever really shown any safe, long-term, sustainable benefits for the average individual who has no dietary derangements or deficiencies in his or her modern choice of foods. Therefore, it's important to weigh the overall risks and the benefits every time you try anything beyond the scope of a safe, natural, earth-grown food.

In a simple, holistic model, a healthy lifestyle should include a balanced diet, a realistic plan to reduce stress, and a moderate exercise routine. Unfortunately, however, people seem to think that this may be a complicated thing. Instead, they are quick to go to extremes to follow anyone that can manage to make a product go viral or succeed in a marketing scheme.

Needless to say, it should be obvious that fad diets are senseless, because the extraordinary results they promise often tend to cause a health and safety mess. The interesting thing is that most people already know this. Yet time and again, they fall for it, only to wake up and once again ask themselves where they went wrong.

For some reason, people think that they can somehow fix their health-related issues with organic diets, vitamins, minerals, or pills. They think they can solve everything with quick-fix cosmetic treatments or elective surgeries.

In light of all the possibilities that have emerged with the modern-day technologies, many have forgotten what the definition of a simple, healthy lifestyle is. In the Western world, many seem to have even lost the ability to determine whether they are really hungry or if they are just craving things.

When it comes to choosing a diet, it's important to remember that balance is the ultimate key. A balanced diet does not necessarily exclude any of the major food groups. What's equally important is that it does not contain an overabundance of factory-processed foods.

A balanced diet simply means consumption in moderation: nothing more, nothing less. It is a simple plan that includes all the elemental nutrients that are deemed essential for proper care and growth of the body but emphasizes moderation and balance as its signature key.

To this end, government websites may serve as a valuable source. When all avenues have failed and all else is exhausted, however, common sense tells me that I can eat anything in moderation, as long as I stick to safe whole foods or naturally processed things. Moreover, before I reach for something, I can't go wrong by asking myself whether I am honestly hungry or if I am just craving things.

Perhaps the most important predictor in achieving and maintaining a healthy lifestyle is an individual's ultimate willingness to stick with the ins and outs of that lifestyle. As with anything worthwhile, a healthy lifestyle needs a lifetime commitment to learn and apply the basic fundamentals that make it work.

Ideally, it may be useful to learn self-imposed, predefined strategies to make sensible decisions when faced with unexpected opportunities to eat. This is especially important if at that moment, one knows that there is no biological need. By setting rules in advance, one may be better equipped to handle one's appetite when faced with that unexpected opportunity to eat.

Even if the food is healthy, there should be no reason to eat or overeat if there is no immediate biological need. Even when sitting at the table, you should learn to consciously recognize whether you really need to eat.

With this understanding, it should be easy to create new eating habits that follow common-sense rules. This simple change will set you free from the bondage of fad diets and yo-yo starvation rules.

Remember, as with anything else, there is no free lunch; if you want results, you need to apply yourself. Help yourself by applying the knowledge and the techniques you've learned in this book.

Use it to make a lasting and profound change in your life. Make it a daily priority to feel good about your conscious choices and eating habits in life. Tastefully picture yourself eating and living your ideal life.

See yourself or, even better, feel yourself maintaining your ideal shape and weight in your ideal healthy state. Use the power of your emotions to affirm your healthy identity and fit state. If you can truly do this with your heart, soul, and brain, you will never have to adopt a restrictive diet again.

THE BOTTOM LINE

Remember, aside from the undeniable benefits of a sensible diet and regular exercise, the most important ingredient in keeping yourself in healthful bliss is the power of your imagination, the power of your mind's creative abyss.

If you were given a glimpse of your body image from the point of view of your subconscious mind, what sort of image do you suppose you would find? On a conscious level, do you like your reflection when you see the mirror image of yourself?

Remember, it's your mind that ultimately dictates how your body responds to the internal or external challenges in your life. Your body by itself is nothing but a vehicle that is ultimately run by your mind.

It's your mind that determines how your body responds to or assimilates your food. The ultimate decision maker is no one else but *you*. Some people eat tons of food and never gain weight, while others manage to put on weight by just dreaming about food.

Could it be that the metabolic conditions you suffer from may simply be the manifestation of the subconscious thoughts and beliefs you have objectified around you? How you see yourself in the mirror and, more importantly, how you mentally perceive your state of health mainly dictate how your body responds to food.

If you say you are weak, ugly, skinny, or fat, then you are right. On the same token, if you hold an ideal picture of your body in your mind, it will do anything within its power to show you are right.

Don't you see that the faulty image you hold of yourself is the very blueprint with which you keep physically creating and re-creating yourself? Wipe away all the mental blemishes or disfiguring deformities you normally see in yourself.

Mentally visualize your body the way you wish to see yourself. If you are not good at visualizing things, then try to feel what it would feel like if you embodied the perfect expression of yourself.

Find healthy role models and try to emulate the attributes and the qualities you admire in them most. Your mind will speedily act to prove your conviction within the boundaries of your own imagination. In other words, *fake it till you make it!* Isn't that what role modeling is all about?

CHAPTER 5

The Esoteric Art of Healing

When faced with an acute injury or a physical trauma, no one in a right mind would even consider thinking twice about trusting the science of Western medicine. But when the ailments become chronic, the general population is bound to encounter an infinite number of alternative therapies and treatment modalities. These may include a wide range of complimentary, hypnotic, holistic, homeopathic, Eastern, tribal, shamanic, or forest- or plant-based practices and recipes.

At times, the options are so overwhelming that it seems

easier to just let someone else take the responsibility of caring for one's well-being. People often want someone else or some higher power to heal them. This, however, is not how things naturally work for mortal beings. If it were, incurable cancers, autoimmune disorders, and chronic conditions would all be cured by someone or something before they have the chance to persist.

The truth is that, in general, people are just unwilling to take responsibility for what they feel they are unfairly experiencing. They just want someone or something to fix everything without having to personally apply themselves or do anything.

Some constantly change doctors in hopes of curing the same nagging thing. What they don't realize is that the power of healing lies not with the doctor but with the inner self, the inner being. They think that the burden of disease is indeed generated from an external source and that they shouldn't be held accountable for anything.

What's amazing is that if you ever catch the slightest glimpse of your inner being, your higher self, you would know without a doubt that everything starts from within. Therefore, the first step in the esoteric art of health and healing is to look inside and let the inward mending process naturally begin. The paradox here, however, is that, though we may call it natural, it should be clear that the process of healing is by no means a passive thing.

The art of health and healing requires a considerable amount of internal discipline. All the examples and the exercises discussed in this book, including using consistent routines that involve emotion, visualization, affirmation, self-love, and kind character are in a way fundamental to the study and practice of the art of health and healing.

It is practically impossible to escape the fact that health is just as much a psychological construct as it is a physical thing. That's why psychology and psychiatry are such broad components of the practice of Western medicine.

To have a healthy, fit, and vibrant body, it is very important that you prepare yourself mentally, just as you do physically in the way of diets and exercises. Remember, the doctor can only do so much. She can help fill her half of the equation, but once she is done, you need to do your part to balance that healing equation.

If you don't do your part in the art of health and healing, you will continue to be prone to the risk of disharmony, pain, disease, and suffering. For this reason, the best time to prepare yourself for health and healing is when you are actually healthy and free from the torments of disease or physical suffering. Therefore, I hope that before you are faced with the inevitable challenges of self-healing, the exercises in this book may help enhance your mental strength and improve your power of healing.

THE ROLE OF BREATHING

Breathing is one of the most essential and consistent life-sustaining functions of the human body. We are literally challenged to involuntarily breathe from the time of birth until the moment we die. Nevertheless, we think nothing of it in terms of its health- or disease-modifying potential in life.

Everyone knows that in the absence of breath, there is no hope; there is no life. What's more, improper breathing can make one more susceptible to premature aging or disease in life.

What most people don't know is that in certain cases, learning the proper mechanics of breathing can help invigorate the body and rejuvenate the rhythm and the flow of life. Long ago, what the sages of the old realized was that though the act of breathing was involuntary, its parameters, including its rate, flow, intensity, and rhythm could be manipulated to optimize its health benefits and therapeutic effects.

The vital force of breathing is intimately intertwined with the vitality of every organ and every system in the body. Therefore, by consciously influencing its rate, rhythm, intensity, and flow, one may be able to enhance its potential to help revitalize and reinvigorate the body and thereby make it constantly regenerate and glow.

Breathing exercises can have a profound effect on the nervous system. Some can help potentially regulate the heartbeat, alter the body's metabolism, and change the threshold of pain. They can affect the processes of digestion, assimilation, and elimination.

They are at times advocated for relaxation, enhanced mood, increased energy, and inner harmony. Some use it to help prevent or alleviate disease. Others use breathing techniques to enhance brain-wave coherence and mental clarity. Some use it as an essential component of meditation. They may even go so far as to call it the secret of spiritual ascension.

Western medicine has scientifically documented the potential benefits of certain breathing patterns in stress management, total body relaxation, insomnia, sleep apnea, and other forms of health and disease management. Incentive spirometers and breathing machines with a variety of adjustable settings are now standards of care in hospital settings and intensive care units.

Some scientists study breathing patterns to demonstrate the power of mind-body connection. Many large medical centers now include the practice of mind-body therapy as an essential part of total care to help prevent or alleviate disease. Some of the therapies offered in these programs inherently incorporate exercises for proper breathing.

The Internet now hosts an extensive body of literature that describes a wide range of breathing patterns for different personalities, different maladies, and different therapies. For example, some involve shallow breathing; others require deep breathing. Some forms entail right- or left-sided breathing techniques through individual nostrils. Others involve complex forms and combinations thereof.

One way or another, many of these exercises aim to invigorate the cells, remove the toxins, and clear or activate the subtle energy channels that are stretched throughout the body. In the end, all these measures are laid out in hopes of promoting health and preventing disease or premature aging.

The caveat, however, is that although breathing exercises can be so incredibly effective, they can be unintentionally dangerous or immanently harmful if mindlessly dabbled in. In fact, in inexperienced hands, they can have a detrimental effect on one's overall health or total well-being.

Therefore, it is best to learn these exercises from a trained expert. When learned from a well-trained and experienced teacher, breathing exercises can help greatly enhance your state of health, balance your psyche, boost your energy, and improve your mental well-being.

THE PLAY OF SENSES

Our sense organs translate the world around us into signals our brains can identify with and understand. In a way, they act like filters in that they tend to only allow recognizable information to pass through. The information they carry to the brain then is decidedly deciphered and processed based on the individual's mind-set, knowledge, expectations, and past experiences.

Depending on one's culture, for example, the sight of a dog may represent a sign of foulness, defilement, fear, pain, or disgust. It may trigger a fight-or-flight response. To another, however, the idea of a dog may represent unconditional devotion, security, love, healing, and trust.

The signals our brains receive from the portals of hearing, touch, taste, smell, and sight get filtered and ultimately translated into the language of pleasure and pain. The interpretation of pleasure and pain, in turn, has the potential to activate physiologic pathways that can either harm the body or flood it with currents of energy, harmony, healing, or love.

We can use this knowledge to create circumstances in which the body can literally heal, grow, and thrive. The idea is to create sensory triggers that are conducive to healing or at least to a vibrant and healthy life. Many spas or health retreats nowadays propose to do just that.

In many of these settings, for example, we are likely to find inviting scenes where we can immerse the mind and body in a sort of a human-made healing spring. They often offer a variety of rejuvenating or healing sense impressions that involve massage therapy, aromatherapy, mineral baths, facials, scrubs, wraps, acupressure, acupuncture, yoga, and healthy dining.

Sadly, for the average individual, many of these venues may seem either impractical or too expensive to take advantage of all year long. At best, they are only visited a few times a year, if even financially or otherwise possible at all. The fact of the matter, however, is that if we want a continuous source of rejuvenation or healing, we need to engage these sensory impressions daily, all year long.

People are more or less familiar with the therapeutic value of a healing touch, a calming scent, or a much-desired taste. Very few, however, pay attention to the healing, regenerating, and rejuvenating benefits of visual or auditory effects.

Normally, we are literally bombarded with a rich supply of visual and auditory information throughout the day. Some of this information is relatively neutral, some can be toxic, while a good portion can be potentially therapeutic and thus beneficial. We can use this knowledge to our advantage to make every day a potentially powerful and healing day. Using the right visual cues and auditory triggers, we can rejuvenate our bodies without the need to take a break or interrupt our day.

THE POWER OF COLOR

Colors can have a profound effect on various layers of consciousness. Why is that important? Because consciousness expresses itself through the physical body; therefore, anything that affects the consciousness also affects the body. Unfortunately, most people are not aware of the inevitable influence colors can potentially exert on the physical body.

It should be no secret that the interplay of light and color can exert a tremendous influence on our moods and feelings. Moods and feelings, in turn, can have a potentially enormous impact on our physical, psychological, and emotional states of being.

Depending on one's personal, social, or cultural orientation, colors can instigate a variety of reactions, moods, and emotions. Certain colors can make you depressed. Some can make you want to go out and buy things. Some colors can promote a sense of happiness. Others may have the potential to elicit a sense of sensuality, tension, or unsolicited violence.

Inarguably, the color arrangements on the walls, the carpets, the furniture, and the accessories in luxurious hotel rooms and lobbies, for example, have a much more relaxing, rejuvenating, and inviting aftereffect, compared to those in a medical or a dental office—don't you agree? Though this may be news to you, the advertisers, interior designers, and the media have successfully capitalized on this knowledge for years. This is one reason why color-conscious hospitals use healing colors, spas use relaxing colors, venues for children's activities use stronger colors, and gambling houses use research-suggested gamblers' colors.

Whether it's to induce a feeling of spaciousness, coziness, happiness, affluence, eroticism, honor, fear, or simple aestheticism, color has long been used to create its corresponding states. Nevertheless, most people walk around in a fog, completely oblivious to the effects colors may have on their moods and conscious states. Colors have a natural tendency to plea to our emotions. Like music, they can set the mood and offer an inviting scene for us to laugh, weep, court, mourn, dance, or ultimately alter our mental, physical, and psychological states.

In a way, the clothes we wear on any given day may ultimately reflect the subtle or not-so-subtle moods we are in that day. The cars we drive, the handbags, the wallets, the shoes, and the accessories we buy all point to an intimate story of our likes and dislikes, unique personalities, and emotional states.

Having noticed all this, then, it should be common sense to think that we can use this knowledge to improve our mental, psychological, and emotional states. We can literally optimize our daily experiences by using our individual color preferences.

To reap the immediate benefits colors may have on our states of consciousness, we do not necessarily need to have them physically on display anywhere in our surrounding space. They can be just as effective in our own imaginations, in our own ideally pictured imaginary universe. In other words, imagining a color is just as effective as seeing it in a real-life display.

In fact, this is actually where all the fun begins. The effect of colors can be just as pronounced and just as substantial when we turn inward and watch an internal scenery of colorful display. In other words, imagining a particular color, with all its vividness, beauty, and splendor, may be just as effective or just as powerful as actually seeing it on a wall, object, or fixture in real life. Ultimately, it's the psychology of color that affects your consciousness, not the physical pigmentation itself.

Let's try a simple mental exercise; go to a quiet room, away from all the disruptions that normally tend to distract you. Lie down in a comfortable position and close your eyes. Try to unwind. Take a few slow deep breaths and relax. Try to relax your body and mind.

Try to imagine yourself naturally floating effortlessly, a few inches above the surface of a warm emerald-green sea. See the dancing impressions on the surface of the water reflecting the shimmering rays of the golden sun. Again, if you can't see anything, then feel it.

Imagine yourself carelessly drifting as you safely absorb the warm rays and feel the healing energy of the sun. Bathe in the healing reflection of that soothing emerald-green color as you absorb the revitalizing energy of that warm spring-day sun.

Imagine the dazzling green and shimmering golden colors permeating, soaking, healing, and revitalizing your body cell by cell. Can you feel this? Take a few slow, deep breaths, come back to the present, and open your eyes. Did you find the colors you generated internally, in your mind's eye, in any way useful or effective?

Now let's try a change of scenery. Make yourself comfortable and close your eyes again. Try to imagine yourself in a warm, wonderfully decorated, cozy room. See yourself feeling safe and comfortable, lying in bed or in front of a fireplace, holding the hands of someone you may intimately know and love. Only this time imagine the room illuminated with an intensely naughty ambient red light.

Feel the wholesome, healthy fire of passion romancing your skin, rising through your spinal column, and flushing your body as you enjoy your evening with the one you love. See yourself cherishing the essence of the intoxicating scent that emanates from the one you love. Imagine yourself deeply immersed in the warmth of that soft, inviting red light. Take a few slow, deep breaths, come back to the present, and open your eyes again. Does the color red in this scenario have any impact on you?

Of course, everyone is different, so finding the best colors or combinations that are specifically right for you may need a little research and tweaking on your part. Maybe the bright light of the sun is the most appropriate color for you. If this is a new concept to you, it may take some time before you can be sure your choice of colors is indeed right for you.

Once you do find the right choice of colors for you, it will become apparent that when you use it in the right context, you may feel a strange sense of harmony in whatever you do. Use the power of colors for health, healing, growth, harmony, or whatever else you may wish to do. Colors can help you get naturally in touch with the inner, healing *you*.

To optimize your use of colors for health and healing, try creating your own mentally assembled, three-dimensional colored or colorful room. Imagine a private place, where you can relax and soak in these colors as you quietly absorb the flow of nature; let this flow rush through your body and utterly cleanse you. Use this room to develop your own source of healing; create your own fountain of vitality and youth.

Try to picture a lasting model of it in your mind and use it regularly to revivify and rejuvenate you. Turn it into an intensely vivid, color-enriched spa or bathing room. Picture yourself bathing in the light of its healing colors as you hover midair in the center of the room. Soak every cell of your body in the healing fabric of this color-filled room.

What colors are healing for you? Create your own colors for energy, vibrancy, vitality, or any other attribute that is desirable for you. Can you see the immense source of vitality you can create for you?

Take a few minutes every day to close your eyes and mentally enter your room. Let it work to regenerate a new *you*. Play in it regularly; visit it often to refresh and revitalize yourself. Do it when you are actually healthy so that you can readily utilize it when you desperately need to nourish and heal yourself.

THE RHYTHM OF SOUND

Every facet of creation in this universe is a form of vibration. Everything in this universe vibrates. The common receptors through which we perceive some of these vibrations happen to be our very own sense organs. Our eyes, noses, ears, tongues, and skin literally help us eavesdrop on the discourse of the universe by sensing its vibrations.

Sound is the brain's narrow perception of a small bandwidth of this vibration. When properly trained, our sense of hearing is said to have the ability to hear the primordial sounds that promote order in this universe. In a way, it has the power to perceive a tiny part of what the cosmos can manifest.

At our current level of conscious evolution, structured sound seems to be our most commonly used method of interpersonal communication. In fact, one might think that without it, we would have a hard time keeping pace with the scales of our creative evolution.

Aside from being an essential vehicle for the purpose of communication, sound is said to be a powerful means of harmony, healing, and spiritual ascension. On the extreme side, it can also serve as a serious form of toxic pollution.

Excessive sounds caused by machines, cars, trucks, trains, aircrafts, factories, and other industrial means are common causes of tension, anxiety, and distress. They are known to increase stress levels, cause sleep disturbances, and account for other potentially serious effects.

Background noise can create distractions, affect creativity, and interfere with one's overall cognitive performance. Artificial noise can cause hearing loss, irritability, impatience, violence, or even physical or psychological imbalance.

On the other hand, sound can be a remarkable source of healing, harmony, and relaxation. It can stir the deepest springs of emotion. It can promote a sense of well-being, euphoria, or relaxation.

Sound is at times used as a powerful means of meditating. Some traditions use it as an integral instrument of healing. Western disciplines use it to image, diagnose, or even treat organs that may be damaged or ailing.

The sound of a chant, prayer, or instrument can at times serve as a potent healing balm. The voice of a child, parent, friend, or a significant other can at times create a feeling of reassurance, consolation, security, and utter calm.

Marching music can move armies across the oceans. It can inspire the masses and mobilize nations. The sound of music can help unite the hopes and dreams of legions. It can either help create violence or spread love and restore harmony among regions or even nations.

Music can be a tremendously potent means of fanning the flames of emotion. That's why singers and musicians can be so influential in the lives of generations.

Music has the power to create the most moving stories and experiences of our lives. It can create chaos or transform one's life into a magical world resembling the Land of Oz. The power of music can help you heal your wounds and change your life.

Many people use music to set the mood and start the day right. Others use it to relax after a long, hard day or night. Many use it to study, to wake up in the morning, or even to fall asleep at night.

Advertisers use music to stir your emotions so you will buy their products. Casinos use it so you will spend your money and tirelessly play. Businesses use it, workplaces use it, restaurants use it; do you get it? The sound of music can easily stir your emotions, and your emotions can easily compel you to act a certain way.

Why not use the emotional power of sound to help you create an energetic, healthy, and vibrant life? Why not use it to cultivate a sense of peace and harmony in your life? Why not use it as an instrument of healing or as a means of purifying and rejuvenating your life?

With the right choice of sound or music, you can consciously create a nurturing environment that is conducive to a state of inner balance, harmony, love, and healing. You can use sound to help you feel energetic and promote a constant sense of well-being.

The Inner Temple of Light

People who accidentally encounter a near-death experience or those who miraculously recover from an accident or a serious illness occasionally report a subjective experience where they may have either traveled through or felt engulfed in an immense body of blinding light. In their descriptions, they often talk about an intimate journey of rejuvenation and healing that took place in the presence of that light.

Why should they feel a sensation of healing in the presence of light? I cannot tell you. It is like trying to find a way around the philosophers "qualia." It's like trying to explain the sensation of pain, the meaning of the color purple, or the aromatic smell of a rose to someone who has never experienced those things before.

How can you explain the healing effect of light to those who have never experienced it this way? To describe its nature or prove its existence is like trying to physically reproduce the images in a dream somehow, someway. It may certainly be possible to show scientific data, suggesting the likelihood that one may have had a dream. But no one can positively verify or re-create the images in that dream. All I can say is that the healing power of light is a dramatic narrative for those who experience it to such extreme.

Whether it's incidental or intentionally induced through visualization, meditation, or otherwise, some people strongly believe that the feeling of bathing in a pool of light is a wonderful supplement to the art of health and healing. Some in fact resort to this sort of remedy long before they choose to seek any form of conventional or alternative therapy.

If you've never heard about this form of healing, you won't know what it can do until you experience it for yourself. It's easy—why not play along and try it for yourself? You have nothing to lose; it can't get any safer than this.

Close your eyes and immerse yourself in an imaginary room that's filled with an intensely bright, life-enhancing light. If you can't visualize the light, then feel what it would feel like if you were engulfed in a body of light. Once again, it's actually the feeling that creates the perceived magic.

Let the light dissolve the impurities of your mind and body cell by cell. Feel the rejuvenating nectar of life penetrate every cell. Let it energize you and fill you with life.

Though for many the practice is always healing and useful, the technique is ideally best learned before one's body is acutely compromised or critically ill. Therefore, it would be much more practical and much more effective if you could make it a simple daily exercise when you are actually healthy and feeling well. Use it regularly to help you feel naturally invigorated and exceptionally well.

Treat yourself to it every day. Use it to relax and rejuvenate yourself after a stressful day. In time, you will begin to experience a blissful, wholesome state that will be readily available for you when you need it night and day. Again, remember, casual attitude and lack of commitment will hardly produce any form of healing that is worthy of use.

CHAPTER 6

Be a Citizen of the Universe

Picture yourself as a single cell among the many trillions that make up the mass of a human body. Imagine being responsible for doing your part in keeping this body in balance and maintaining a sense of harmony. See yourself absorbing nutrients, regulating waste, replacing your worn-out parts, engulfing microorganisms, disarming intruders, subduing foreign invaders, and sending or receiving messages to and from other cells.

Picture yourself having the ability to release substances that nourish and nurture the surrounding cells. See yourself working with other cells to ensure overall synchrony and total body harmony. In sum, see yourself serving the body by doing your part to keep it happy and healthy.

True, one cell, in the midst of the many trillions, seems so weak and inconsequential. Yet, it possesses the power to cause enough damage to destroy regions, paralyze organs, weaken limbs, or even affect the entire body.

What would happen if someday you suddenly decided to stage a mutiny? What would happen if someday you suddenly decided to single-handedly rebel against the body? Though you may be only a single cell, wouldn't you become antagonistic to the entire body?

You could release poisonous substances, for example, that have the potential to cause tissue damage or disturb the process of normal growth. You could send erroneous signals and trick other cells into mobilizing an immune response. By doing this, you can even potentially start an inflammatory response.

If you think about it for a moment, you could see how your single-cell rebellion has the potential to ultimately trigger a toxic response. It could lead to local necrosis or, even worse yet, organ damage or an adverse systemic response.

You could replicate out of control and interfere with the body's natural and orderly growth. You can transform yourself into a cancer cell and cause uninhibited growth.

Alternatively, what would happen if you chose to nurture and nourish the body? You would ensure proper conduct and self-regulation. You would try to do your part in establishing a sense of balance and total harmony.

You would try to live in peace and respect your

neighboring cells. You would synchronize your efforts with all the other cells. You would bathe the surrounding cells in fortifying substances. You would do your best to trigger happy signals for other cells.

In many ways, one can argue that you, as a mere individual in this lonely corner of the cosmos, possess potential qualities that are strikingly similar to those of a single cell. Hypothetically, you are an isolated being in the midst of all the billions, with seemingly insignificant influence yet infinite potential power to affect everything.

You as an individual can give birth to new life. You have the power to move mountains, destroy worlds, and explore the distant corners of the universe. You can fly in the air, dive deep into the mysterious seas, and travel into the void realm of space.

As a human being, you have the ability to take advantage of many of the fundamental laws of nature. You can overcome gravity, direct electricity, use the magnetic field, communicate wirelessly, and change the Earth's ecological balance to suit your needs.

You possess the potential power to start a human revolution all by yourself. You can change trends, create the future, and lead the masses. You can start constructive endeavors with unified aims and ideals that can change the direction and the destiny of the human race.

It's all up to you. You have the power to work against the body of the universe. You can cause significant harm and destroy things. You can stay stationary and simply eke out a mere life of marginal existence and misery.

You can choose to be a lead weight on the shoulders of all those who carry the torch of victory. You can be the mist that obscures the road to innovation and prosperity.

Alternatively, you can strive to make this world a better place by spreading the seeds of love, joy, and harmony. You can be a beacon of love, a composer of a happy symphony. You can be a messenger of peace and virtue for all of humanity.

You can heal people and touch others in ways that can be felt for centuries. You can be a lighthouse of goodness and honor that lights up all the dark places on Earth and changes people's destinies. Which would you choose? One way or another, the choice is yours.

This world is a playground created solely for *you*, for you to express yourself through the creativity, brilliance, and the ingenuity that are part and parcel of *you*. This playground is created for you to discover your supreme mastery over all the forces that try to suppress the freedom and the powers that are inherently dormant within you.

You have the power to rule over it all, not through automatic heirship, mind you, but through uncovering, unearthing, and unlocking all the mysterious laws of nature that miraculously surround you. Everything you see around you, every blade of grass, every molecule of air, every drop of water, every animal, every seemingly inanimate object, every moon, every planet, every star, and every galaxy literally exists for no one else but you.

Everything you see around yourself demands your claim of mastery and ownership, not by force, but by igniting the spark of that inner fire within you. You are the creator of the universe; you are the rightful heir to this vast dominion; you are the centerpiece in the totality of the aggregate that makes up the whole cosmos.

All the languages, all the ancient writings, and all the wisdom of history are at your disposal. All the good things in life are here to fortify you. All the human beings on this Earth are here to help you. All the animals, all the creatures, all the organisms, all the solid objects, all the mountains, seas, stars, and skies are here to give you a nudge and provide clues.

All the visual wonders, all the sounds, and the scents of nature exist to fortify you. Won't you at least try to see your potential within this powerful universal scheme that's created for you? If you don't see it, you have no one else to blame but *you*. Set out on the road to self-discovery. The path is open; won't you allow yourself to walk through?

Like a balloon-bound measure of air that finally bursts through the elastic walls and realizes its oneness with the totality of the atmosphere, try to become conscious of your status as the sole creator of your universe. Be a befitting deity; try to realize your oneness with this universe.

You are the creator, the created, and the force of creation that sustains us all. You come from that same source of life that is shared by us all. Therefore, love everyone, wish goodness for everyone, and offer your heart and your blessings to everyone. After all, we are all but simple expressions of the *one*.

Once you realize your oneness with the all, you will begin to feel the peace and the harmony that this world shares with us all. When you are finally in tune with the harmony that underlies all, you will begin to enjoy the health, the vitality, and the energy that inwardly belong to us all.

About the Author

HOMAYOUN SADEGHI, M.D. is an innovative modern-day physician. His new book, The Art of Healthy Living: A Mind-Body Approach to Inner Balance and Natural Vitality is receiving critical and popular acclaim as a simple and eloquent work that changes lives and opens the mind to new possibilities. He has authored and published abstracts and articles that are widely quoted and cited in prominent national and international scientific journals.

As a mind-body expert, educator, and speaker, Dr. Sadeghi is an advocate of combining the needs of modern living with the power of insight, intuition, wisdom, and inner healing. He believes that a healthy body starts from the inside out. Dr. Sadeghi embraces a holistic approach and stresses the importance of a well-balanced mind and body in the art of well-being. To this end, he emphasizes the intimate role of consciousness in creating and influencing the nature of the body — and ultimately our physical reality.

www.SadeghiMD.com

I hope you enjoyed this book.
To learn more or for information on upcoming books
and events, please go to **www.SadeghiMD.com**

Made in the USA
San Bernardino, CA
01 September 2016